Your Child with Inflammatory Bowel Disease

A Johns Hopkins Press Health Book

Your Child with Inflammatory Bowel Disease

A Family Guide for Caregiving

SECOND EDITION

North American Society for Pediatric
Gastroenterology, Hepatology and Nutrition

EDITORS-IN-CHIEF

Maria Oliva-Hemker, MD

David Ziring, MD

Shehzad A. Saeed, MD

Athos Bousvaros, MD, MPH

Johns Hopkins University Press
Baltimore

Johns Hopkins University Press
2715 North Charles Street
Baltimore, Maryland 21218-4363
www.press.jhu.edu

Library of Congress Cataloging-in-Publication Data

Names: Oliva-Hemker, Maria, editor. | Ziring, David, editor. | Saeed, Shehzad A.,
    editor. | Bousvaros, Athos, editor.
Title: Your child with inflammatory bowel disease : a family guide for
    caregiving / North American Society for Pediatric Gastroenterology,
    Hepatology and Nutrition ; editors-in-chief Maria Oliva-Hemker, MD, David
    Ziring, MD, Shehzad A. Saeed, MD, Athos Bousvaros, MD, MPH.
Description: Second edition. | Baltimore : Johns Hopkins University Press,
    [2017] | Series: A Johns Hopkins Press health book | Includes
    bibliographical references and index.
Identifiers: LCCN 2017007356| ISBN 9781421423517 (pbk. : alk. paper) | ISBN
    1421423510 (pbk. : alk. paper) | ISBN 9781421423524 (electronic) | ISBN
    1421423529 (electronic)
Subjects: LCSH: Inflammatory bowel diseases—Popular works. | Gastroenteritis
    in children—Popular works. | Caregivers—Popular works.
Classification: LCC RJ456.G3 Y68 2017 | DDC 618.92/33—dc23
    LC record available at https://lccn.loc.gov/2017007356

All illustrations are by Jacqueline Schaffer.

Special discounts are available for bulk purchases of this book. For more information, please contact Special Sales at 410-516-6936 or specialsales@press.jhu.edu.

Johns Hopkins University Press uses environmentally friendly book materials, including recycled text paper that is composed of at least 30 percent post-consumer waste, whenever possible.

The facing page is an extension of this copyright page.

Contents

Contributors

Susan S. Baker, MD, PhD
  Children's Hospital of Buffalo
  Buffalo, New York

Robert N. Baldassano, MD*
  Children's Hospital of
    Philadelphia
  Philadelphia, Pennsylvania

Keith J. Benkov, MD*
  The Mount Sinai Hospital
  New York, New York

Athos Bousvaros, MD
  Children's Hospital
  Boston, Massachusetts

Jeffrey B. Brown, MD
  Children's Memorial Hospital
  Chicago, Illinois

Steven Brown, MBBS, PhD
  Mount Sinai School of Medicine
  New York, New York

Mitchell B. Cohen, MD
  Cincinnati Children's Hospital
    Medical Center
  Cincinnati, Ohio

Stanley A. Cohen, MD
  Children's Center for Digestive
    Healthcare
  Atlanta, Georgia

Richard B. Colletti, MD
  University of Vermont
  Burlington, Vermont

Wallace V. Crandall, MD
  Nationwide Children's Hospital
  Columbus, Ohio

Karen Denise Crissinger, MD, PhD
  University of South Alabama
  Mobile, Alabama

Carmen Cuffari, MD
  The Johns Hopkins Children's
    Center
  Baltimore, Maryland

Fredric Daum, MD
  Winthrop University Hospital
  New York, New York

Marla Dubinsky, MD
  The Mount Sinai Hospital
  New York, New York

Adi R. Ferrara**
  Bellevue, Washington

George D. Ferry, MD
  Texas Children's Hospital
  Houston, Texas

Benjamin Gold, MD
  Children's Center for Digestive
    Healthcare
  Atlanta, Georgia

Anne M. Griffiths, MD*
  Hospital for Sick Children
  Toronto, Ontario, Canada

Sandeep Gupta, MD
  Riley Hospital for Children
  Indianapolis, Indiana

Melvin B. Heyman, MD, MPH
  San Francisco Children's Hospital
  San Francisco, California

Leslie M. Higuchi, MD
  Children's Hospital
  Boston, Massachusetts

Jeffrey S. Hyams, MD*
  Connecticut Children's Medical
    Center
  Hartford, Connecticut

Mark J. Integlia, MD
  Cape Elizabeth, Maine

David M. Israel, MD, FRCP
  British Columbia Children's
    Hospital
  Vancouver, British Columbia,
    Canada

Esther Israel, MD
  Massachusetts General Hospital
  Boston, Massachusetts

Robert M. Issenman, MD
  McMaster Children's Hospital
  Hamilton, Ontario, Canada

Howard A. Kader, MD
  University of Maryland Medical
    Center
  Baltimore, Maryland

Marsha Kay, MD
  Cleveland Clinic Foundation
  Cleveland, Ohio

David J. Keljo, MD, PhD
  University of Pittsburgh School
    of Medicine
  Pittsburgh, Pennsylvania

Barbara S. Kirschner, MD
  University of Chicago Children's
    Hospital
  Chicago, Illinois

Alan M. Leichtner, MD
  Children's Hospital
  Boston, Massachusetts

David R. Mack, MD
  Children's Hospital of Eastern
    Ontario
  Ottawa, Ontario, Canada

Laura Mackner
  Nationwide Children's Hospital
  Columbus, Ohio

Lori Mahajan, MD
Cleveland Clinic Foundation
Cleveland, Ohio

Petar Mamula, MD
Children's Hospital of
Philadelphia
Philadelphia, Pennsylvania

James F. Markowitz, MD*
North Shore–LIJ Health System
New Hyde Park, New York

Jonathan E. Markowitz, MD
Greenville Children's Hospital
Greenville, South Carolina

Adelina McDuffie, RN, MS, CPNP
Children's Hospital of Kings
Daughters
Norfolk, Virginia

Mary Susan Moyer, MD
Cincinnati Children's Hospital
Medical Center
Cincinnati, Ohio

Maria Oliva-Hemker, MD
The Johns Hopkins Children's
Center
Baltimore, Maryland

Anthony Otley, MD
IWK Health Centre
Halifax, Nova Scotia, Canada

Susan Peck, RN, MSN, CPNP
Children's Hospital of
Philadelphia
Philadelphia, Pennsylvania

David A. Piccoli, MD
Children's Hospital of
Philadelphia
Philadelphia, Pennsylvania

D. Brent Polk, MD
Children's Hospital Los Angeles
Los Angeles, California

Joel R. Rosh, MD
Morristown Memorial Hospital
Morristown, New Jersey

Gary J. Russell, MD
Massachusetts General Hospital
Boston, Massachusetts

Shehzad Saeed, MD
Dayton Children's Health Partners
Dayton, Ohio

Bruce Sands, MD
Massachusetts General Hospital
Boston, Massachusetts

Judy B. Splawski, MD
Rainbow Babies and Children's
Hospital
Cleveland, Ohio

Maya D. Srivastava, MD, PhD
Center for Digestive, Allergic and
Immunologic Diseases
Williamsville, New York

Michael C. Stephens, MD
Medical College of Wisconsin
Milwaukee, Wisconsin

Francisco Sylvester, MD
University of North Carolina
Children's Hospital
Chapel Hill, North Carolina

Eva Szigethy, MD
University of Pittsburgh
Pittsburgh, Pennsylvania

Vasundhara Tolia, MD
Children's Hospital of Michigan
Detroit, Michigan

William R. Treem, MD
Children's Hospital at Downstate
Brooklyn, New York

John N. Udall, Jr., MD, PhD
West Virginia University
Charleston, West Virginia

Eric Vasiliauskas, MD
Cedars-Sinai Medical Center
Los Angeles, California

Menno Verhave, MD
Children's Hospital
Boston, Massachusetts

Steven L. Werlin, MD
Medical College of Wisconsin
Milwaukee, Wisconsin

Harland S. Winter, MD*
Massachusetts General Hospital
for Children
Boston, Massachusetts

Robert Wyllie, MD
Cleveland Clinic Foundation
Cleveland, Ohio

David Ziring, MD
Cedars-Sinai Medical Center
Los Angeles, California

* Founding Editor
** Medical Writer and Editor

Preface

The first time I heard the phrase "Crohn's disease," I was about 5 years old. I didn't know what it was, but I knew this: Crohn's disease was the reason my mom was in the hospital and not home with me. My sister was diagnosed when she was 9. I was diagnosed when I was 13 years old. Crohn's disease was the norm at my house. I was curious about this disease that was affecting most of my family, and I bombarded my doctors with questions:

> Was I going to have to be in the hospital like my mom?
> Would I have the disease forever?
> Why do so many people in my family have Crohn's disease?

Their answers only fueled my curiosity. I needed to understand more. I can't be positive, but I am fairly certain that my diagnosis of Crohn's disease led me to medical school and, eventually, to become a pediatric gastroenterologist.

My knowledge of inflammatory bowel disease (IBD) has grown exponentially since I was first diagnosed. I have learned from books and journals, from my own experiences as a patient, and from the patients with IBD whom I care for. I have learned that no one person's illness is exactly the same as another person's. I have learned that some people can eat anything, and some people are sensitive to foods. The most difficult lesson I've learned is that despite my best efforts, I cannot predict my disease or the disease of my patients.

I have found that understanding my disease and IBD in general has helped me as a patient. It is important to recognize symptoms and what they can mean, why things happen, and how medications work. I believe that the more patients and families understand these issues, the more likely they are to take their medications and to seek help early when problems develop.

While I wouldn't wish the diagnosis of IBD on anyone, I can honestly say that Crohn's disease has made me a better person. I have gained perspective. I have learned what's important. I have had the privilege of watching children with IBD grow up and follow their dreams. These children inspire me. I have met architects, teachers, a professional golfer, a NASCAR driver, a professional hockey coach, an Iron Man athlete, and countless others with IBD. I have learned that having IBD isn't fun, but that it doesn't stop you from succeeding at anything you set your mind to do.

This book is the second edition of a fantastic resource for patients and families. Its purpose is to provide the foundation of your IBD education, not to substitute for discussion with your child's doctor. The book provides reliable information about the importance of symptoms, the role of tests and studies, and the options for treatment, as well as help satisfying your curiosity about the disease. Writing this book was a labor of love by a team of physicians who care deeply for their patients and appreciate the role of knowledge as a part of treatment. My family and I would have appreciated having the insight and resources found in this book throughout our experiences with IBD.

Cheryl Blank, DO
Pediatric Gastroenterologist
Maine Medical Center, Portland, Maine

Acknowledgments

This book reflects the hard work of more than fifty experts, each of whom wrote a section of the book that was then integrated into the whole. The project was started years ago by a team of physicians who solicited contributions from members of the North American Society for Pediatric Gastroenterology, Hepatology and Nutrition. Those doctors are each designated as a "founding editor" (with an asterisk) in the list of contributors. The manuscript was revised by Adi Ferrara, a medical writer. The physicians who became the editors-in-chief then updated the content, added new sections, and rewrote the book extensively to give it one voice. The wonderful team at Johns Hopkins University Press performed the final revising, editing, and illustrating.

Because this book has been extensively rewritten, we cannot assign authorship of a specific chapter to any individual or group of individuals. This book should therefore be considered a team effort by all the people listed as contributing authors. If we have inadvertently omitted any contributor during this process, we apologize.

We would like to dedicate this book to the memory of Susan Moyer, a caring and kind physician who spent her life improving the health of children with Crohn's disease and ulcerative colitis.

Part I
About IBD

1

An Overview of Inflammatory Bowel Disease

If you are reading this book, your child has likely been diagnosed with a form of inflammatory bowel disease. If your child has been diagnosed recently, many questions may be running through your mind:

Why does my child have this condition? What caused it?
Is it serious?
How is it treated?
What should my child eat?

This part of the book describes the healthy digestive system, and it explains how inflammatory bowel disease causes digestive problems. Later chapters answer many other questions you may have. You will probably have still more questions after reading this book; if you do, the resources listed in chapter 22 may help. Don't forget, though, that your health care team should be your primary source for medical knowledge about your child's illness.

What Is IBD?

Inflammatory bowel disease (IBD) is a general term that usually refers to one of three different conditions: Crohn's disease (CD), ulcerative colitis (UC), and indeterminate colitis (IC). Indeterminate colitis, or inflammatory bowel disease unclassified (IBDU), is a term used to describe IBD when physicians cannot determine whether the person has CD or UC, though a diagnosis of one or the other often becomes clearer over time.

Crohn's disease and ulcerative colitis have some genetic differences, can affect different portions of the intestine, and are sometimes treated differently. Yet they share enough features to be grouped under the name *inflammatory bowel disease*. IBD causes inflammation (swelling and irritation) somewhere in the digestive system, most commonly in the large intestine (the *colon*). IBD can also cause problems outside the digestive system.

The inflammation of IBD occurs when a person's immune cells attack his own digestive system (the gastrointestinal, or GI, tract). The immune cells are the cells that normally clear bacteria and other disease-causing organisms from the body. Why does the body attack its own GI

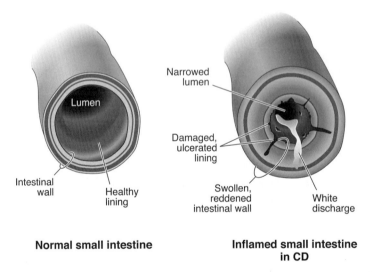

Normal small intestine

Inflamed small intestine in CD

Figure 1.1. Cross-sectional views of normal and inflamed small intestine. The intestine looks like a hollow tube. Food and liquid pass through the center of the tube (the *intestinal lumen*). As nutrients pass, they are broken down and absorbed on the inner surface of the intestine (the *mucosa*, or inner lining). The wall of the intestine is normally thin (*left*). When the intestine is inflamed, as in Crohn's disease (*right*), the wall of the intestine becomes thickened and red, and the lumen may become narrow.

tract? Research suggests that IBD occurs when a person inherits genes that make him susceptible to IBD and is then exposed to something in the environment that makes his intestine's immune system react against the bowel (figure 1.1). When inflammation occurs, the intestine becomes red and swollen.

Researchers have not yet isolated all the genes involved in CD or UC. They have also not discovered which specific environmental factors trigger the diseases. Nonetheless, research into inheritance and environment has made great progress in the past twenty years. Physicians and scientists hope that with ongoing study, we will be able to identify the causes of CD and UC. Research is continuing in these areas.

We return to the discussion of UC and CD near the end of this chapter. First, though, we briefly review the structure and functions of the GI tract and explore why the intestine is so important to human health, what *inflammation* means, and what happens when the intestine becomes inflamed.

What Is the Gastrointestinal Tract, and What Does It Do?

Structure and Functions of the Digestive System

The primary roles of the gastrointestinal tract (or digestive system) are to convert food into simple substances that can be used by the body as energy and to eliminate waste. Food is composed of three main substances: carbohydrates (sugars and starches), proteins, and fats (lipids). The digestive system takes food, grinds it, and breaks it down into *building blocks*, including simple sugars, amino acids, and fatty acids. These building blocks can be absorbed by intestinal cells, delivered to the bloodstream, and used by the different organs of the body, including the heart, lungs, brain, and muscles. If the intestine doesn't function properly, the body can't digest food well, and the person is at risk of developing malnutrition (lack of calories and energy).

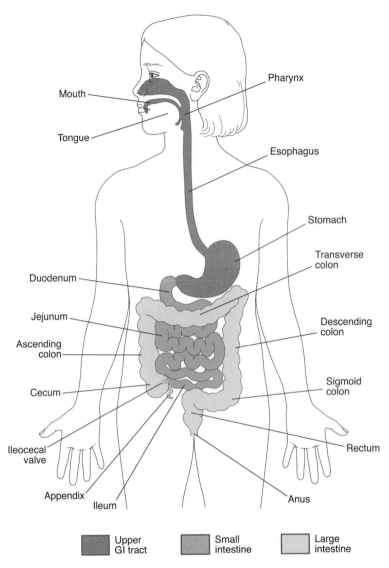

Figure 1.2. Map of the digestive system. Food starts in the mouth, passes through the esophagus, then into the stomach and the first part of the small intestine (*duodenum*). The second part of the small intestine is the *jejunum*, and the lower part is the *ileum*. Digested intestinal contents leaving the small intestine enter the first part of the large intestine, or *cecum*. They then pass through the ascending colon, transverse colon, descending colon, sigmoid colon, and rectum before being expelled.

The gastrointestinal tract consists of different segments (figure 1.2). The mouth and *pharynx* (throat) swallow food and deliver it to the esophagus, a long tube that carries food from the mouth to the stomach. The stomach is a powerful muscle whose main purpose is to mechanically grind food into small pieces (food particles). Once the food particles are sufficiently small, they pass into the small intestine. The small intestine can be thought of as a very long, flexible tube or cylinder—in the average adult, the length of the small intestine is approximately 18 to 20 feet. The inner portion of the cylinder, where food, fluid, and digestive juices are located, is called the *lumen*.

The main purpose of the small intestine is to absorb food and water. Once food particles enter the small intestine, the particles mix with intestinal fluid and digestive juices from the liver and pancreas. Here, in the intestinal lumen, foods are broken down into their building blocks. Specifically, starches are broken down into simple sugars, proteins are broken down into amino acids, and fats are broken down into fatty acids and *monoglycerides*. At this point, foods are ready to be absorbed by the small intestinal lining (*intestinal epithelium*).

The cells of the small intestinal lining can be seen only with a microscope. The most common cell in the intestinal lining is the intestinal absorptive cell (the *enterocyte*); billions of these cells line the intestine. They are specially designed to transport the nutritional building blocks (sugars, amino acids, and fatty acids) into the bloodstream. To improve digestion, these cells are positioned in fingerlike projections called *villi*. Thus, the inner surface of the small intestine is not flat but is composed of thousands and thousands of little "intestinal fingers" that help absorb food. Healthy villi can be seen by the gastroenterologist with a high-magnification endoscope or under a microscope (figure 1.3).

The small intestine gradually pushes food particles down the length of its 18 or so feet to the *ileocecal valve*. (The valve is like a doorway between the small intestine and the large intestine.) By the time food particles leave the small intestine, most of their nutritional value has been extracted, and what is left is the waste, or undigested food (roughage). What enters the large intestine (colon) is a mushy brown fluid. The main role of the large

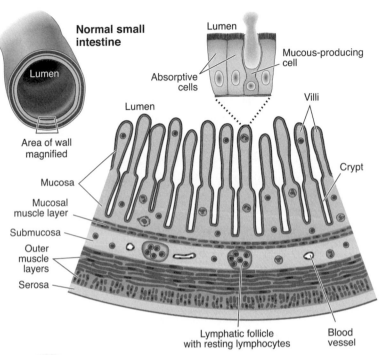

Normal small intestine

Lumen

Mucous-producing cell

Absorptive cells

Lumen

Villi

Crypt

Area of wall magnified

Mucosa

Mucosal muscle layer

Submucosa

Outer muscle layers

Serosa

Lymphatic follicle with resting lymphocytes

Blood vessel

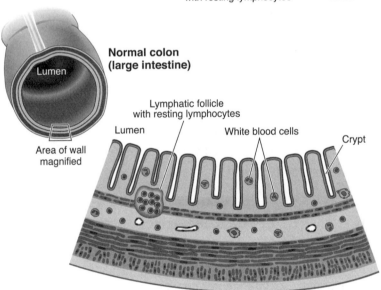

Normal colon (large intestine)

Lumen

Lymphatic follicle with resting lymphocytes

White blood cells

Lumen

Crypt

Area of wall magnified

intestine is to further thicken the stool by absorbing water from the stool back into the body. Thus, the stool that comes out of the anus is usually formed. Although the colon is useful in preventing dehydration, one does not need the colon to absorb food, and people can maintain their weight and hydration without a colon if they eat and drink enough.

The Intestine's Immune System

Another role of the intestine is to protect against infections. Every day, the intestine is exposed to "invaders" from outside our bodies. These invaders include the bacteria and viruses we swallow after inhaling them through our nose, bacteria in the soil and ground, and the organisms that live in contaminated food and drinking water. To protect from infection, the intestine has an elaborate immune system. This system is not an organ like the heart or gut but a collective name for cells that travel around the body. The best-known cells of the immune system are the white blood cells, which can be found in both the blood and the tissues (for example, the lungs and the gut). These immune system cells (white blood cells and others) live in the different layers of the intestine. The main purpose of the intestine's immune system is to prevent bacteria and viruses from entering the bloodstream and doing damage throughout the body. If the

Figure 1.3. Magnified views of the lining of the small intestine and the colon, showing villi and immune system cells. In the small intestine, the absorptive and mucous cells lining the inner layer (*inset, top*) are arranged in fingerlike structures called *villi*. The villi help increase surface area for absorption of food. Below the villi are *crypts*, which secrete intestinal fluid. Underneath the innermost layer (*mucosa*) is another layer (*submucosa*), which includes blood vessels (for absorption of digested nutrients) and cells of the immune system (*lymphatic follicles*). Underneath the mucosa and submucosa are muscle layers that can contract and push food through the intestine.

The colon (large intestine) has a structure similar to the structure of the small intestine. However, because the colon is not as important as the small intestine in absorbing digested food and nutrients, its surface is flat, without villi.

cells of the immune system are inappropriately turned on, or *activated*, however, they have the potential to damage the person's own intestine.

What Does Inflammation Mean?

The word *inflammation* comes from the Latin word *inflamatio*, which means literally "to set on fire." The term is attributed to Aulus Cornelius Celsus, a Roman physician, who described the four characteristics of infected tissues: pain, redness, swelling, and warmth. An easily understood example of inflammation is a streptococcal throat infection (strep throat). In strep throat, a bacterial infection causes the throat to be red (inflamed) and sore, and may cause the throat to produce a whitish discharge (pus). Similarly, the colon or small intestine in CD or UC may be red and sore, with mucus and a white discharge (called *exudate*). Looking at inflamed tissue under the microscope, the physician sees many white blood cells.

In bacterial infections, such white blood cells are helpful in clearing the infection, but at times inflammation can be harmful. Harmful inflammation occurs when the body's immune system attacks the body's own tissues; a condition that causes this process is often called an *autoimmune*, or *autoinflammatory*, disease. Examples of such illnesses include diabetes (where the immune system attacks the pancreas), psoriasis (where the immune system attacks the skin), rheumatoid arthritis (where the immune system attacks the joints), and inflammatory bowel disease (where the immune system attacks the intestine). In ulcerative colitis, the pain, redness, and swelling are limited to the large intestine (colon). In Crohn's disease, the inflammation can occur not only in the colon, but also in the small intestine and other areas of the gastrointestinal tract.

What Is Ulcerative Colitis?

Ulcerative colitis (UC) is a type of inflammatory bowel disease in which inflammation is usually found only in the large intestine. Two English physicians, Samuel Wilks and Walter Moxon, are credited with describing UC in 1875 as a condition different from diarrheal diseases caused by infectious agents. The term *ulcerative* is used because small breaks, called ulcers, can be seen in the lining of the colon when the disease is active, and these can cause the person to have symptoms. Ulcers are areas where the lining of the intestine has been so damaged that it has been worn away, leaving a sore. Shallow ulcers commonly occur in the large intestine in active ulcerative colitis. *Colitis* means inflammation (-itis) of the large intestine (colon). In children, UC usually involves the entire colon (*pancolitis*). In some children, however, the colitis affects only the left side of the colon (*left-sided colitis*), or the very end of the colon—the rectum (*ulcerative proctitis*) (figure 1.4).

The symptoms of ulcerative colitis—such as diarrhea, rectal bleeding, and abdominal pain—result directly from inflammation of the large intestine. UC symptoms vary over time. When a patient is having cramps, diarrhea, and rectal bleeding, she is usually experiencing what is called a *flare*, an *exacerbation*, or a period of *active disease*. In contrast, when a patient feels well and has no significant digestive symptoms, she is considered to be in *remission*. In addition to gut symptoms, people with IBD may also develop inflammation outside their GI tract, such as joint swelling (*arthritis*), eye redness (*uveitis*), or skin rashes. IBD complications that occur in organs other than the intestine are called *extraintestinal symptoms*. These symptoms are discussed in more detail in chapter 12.

Although UC is a lifelong illness, it can usually be well controlled with medications. One or more than one medication may be used during flares (periods of disease activity) or during periods of remission. Patients usually need to be treated with medications even if they are in remission because medications can be used to prevent disease flares. These medications are sometimes called *maintenance therapies* because they are used to maintain the GI tract in a healthy state. The course of UC is also variable; some people have more frequent flares than others. In a small number of people, the disease does not respond well to medications, and surgical options may need to be considered (see chapter 11).

In summary, ulcerative colitis is a disease characterized by a typical pattern of inflammation in the large intestine. The most common symp-

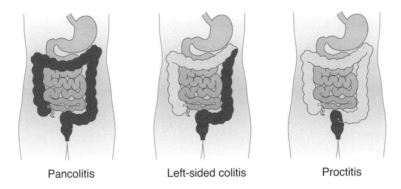

Pancolitis   Left-sided colitis   Proctitis

Common locations for ulcerative colitis

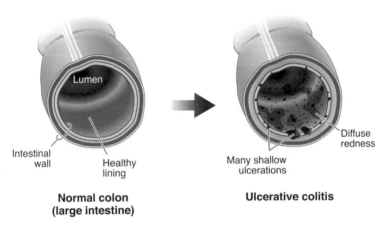

Normal colon   **Ulcerative colitis**
(large intestine)

Figure 1.4. Common locations for ulcerative colitis. The inflammation in ulcerative colitis is usually limited to the large intestine (colon). In most children, the entire colon is inflamed (pancolitis; *top left*). In about 25 percent of children, only the left side of the colon is affected (left-sided colitis; *middle*). In less than 10 percent of children, the inflammation is limited to the rectum (proctitis; *top right*). The inflammation in ulcerative colitis is characterized by a change in the normal colon's healthy lining (*bottom left*), making that inner lining red and ulcerated (*bottom right*).

toms during a flare are abdominal cramping, diarrhea, and rectal bleeding. The physician and the parent share the same goal: to control the child's illness so that flares are as short as possible and remissions are as long as possible.

What Is Crohn's Disease?

Crohn's disease (CD) is similar to ulcerative colitis in that it causes inflammation of the intestines. The main difference between CD and UC is the area of intestine most commonly involved. The disease in UC is limited to the large intestine. In contrast, CD can occur in any part of the GI tract, between the mouth and the anus. The most common places are the last portion of the small intestine (the *terminal ileum*) and the first part of the large intestine (the *cecum*). Crohn's disease was first described in 1932 by three physicians, Burrill Crohn, Leon Ginzberg, and Gordon Oppenheimer.

A second major difference between CD and UC is that the inflammation in CD is often deeper and involves the whole wall of the colon or the small intestine (*transmural inflammation*). The severity of the inflammation can vary from tiny ulcers to large, deep, and destructive ulcers. Most of the time, the ulcers are small and heal easily with medication. Sometimes, though, a deep ulcer forms a hole in the intestine, which leads to an abdominal infection, called an *abscess* (figure 1.5). The abdominal abscess occurs because a hole in the intestine allows intestinal fluid to leak into the cavity of the abdomen. Inflammation in CD can also cause an area of the bowel to be narrowed, or *strictured*, which can partially obstruct the passage of digestive fluids and air through the GI tract and cause cramps and vomiting.

Crohn's disease, like ulcerative colitis, is characterized by active periods of symptoms (flares) alternating with inactive periods when the person is feeling well (remission). But the symptoms of CD may differ from the symptoms of UC. Because Crohn's sometimes involves the small intestine but not the large intestine, people with CD often have belly pain, fatigue, and weight loss without rectal bleeding. As with UC, the primary treatment for CD is medication, and the common aim of the physician and parent is to keep flares as short as possible and remission as long as possible. In addition to medication, some people might benefit from dietary therapy (see chapter 13), while others might benefit from surgery to remove a portion of the diseased intestine (chapter 11).

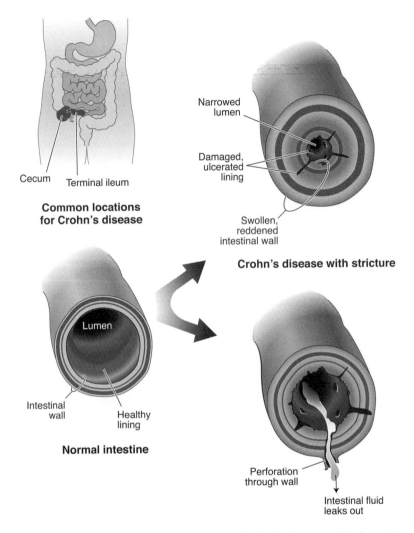

Common locations for Crohn's disease

Cecum

Terminal ileum

Crohn's disease with stricture

Narrowed lumen

Damaged, ulcerated lining

Swollen, reddened intestinal wall

Normal intestine

Lumen

Intestinal wall

Healthy lining

Crohn's disease with abscess

Perforation through wall

Intestinal fluid leaks out

Figure 1.5. Crohn's disease can involve any region of the intestine, but the most common area is the last part of the small intestine (the terminal ileum) and the first part of the large intestine (the cecum). Over time, the inflammation may result in different complications. Some patients may develop a thick intestinal wall and a narrow lumen (a stricture; *top right*), which results in an inability to pass food through the intestine (obstruction). Other patients with Crohn's may develop a hole in the intestinal wall (perforation), resulting in leakage of intestinal fluid into the abdomen (abdominal abscess; *bottom right*).

What Is Indeterminate Colitis?

At times, after a gastroenterologist has thoroughly tested a patient, the physician cannot tell whether the IBD is Crohn's disease or ulcerative colitis. This usually occurs when the person has IBD that involves the large intestine (like UC) but also has some features that suggest CD. These patients may be given a diagnosis of *indeterminate colitis* (IC), also known as *inflammatory bowel disease unclassified* (IBDU). Often patients with IC are treated very much like patients with UC, then reevaluated later to see if their disease can now be called either Crohn's or ulcerative colitis.

So your child's diagnosis of IBD may be subdivided into one of three main groups: ulcerative colitis, Crohn's disease, or indeterminate colitis. Once diagnosed, most people with IBD can be treated with medications to get the disease under control and to keep them feeling well (see chapter 10). Most children respond well to treatment and can lead a normal life. All children with IBD, however, need long-term follow-up with a gastroenterology team for medical treatment, nutritional assessments, and emotional support.

回 2

IBD Causes and Risk Factors

Inflammatory bowel disease has been a topic of study by doctors and scientists for more than fifty years, but we still do not know precisely what causes IBD or why some people develop it. Scientists believe that both genetics and the environment play major roles in the development of the disease. The interaction between genes and the environment most likely activates (turns on) the cells of the immune system, causing the intestinal symptoms. This chapter will summarize what we know and what we don't know about possible causes of IBD. We are optimistic that future research will help us pinpoint the causes of these mysterious illnesses.

The Epidemiology of IBD

The term *epidemiology* refers to the study of disease distribution and frequency. Epidemiologists are scientists who ask questions such as these:

Who gets a disease?
How common is the disease?
Are there any factors that put a person at risk for getting the disease?

Epidemiologists have concluded, for example, that smokers have a greater risk of lung cancer than nonsmokers, and that African Americans are at higher risk for developing sickle cell disease than are Caucasians.

Epidemiologists estimate that more than 1.5 million people living in the United States have IBD. Thus, IBD affects 1 in every 300 Americans. Approximately 100,000 of those Americans with IBD are children. More than 3 million Europeans have IBD. Studies from both the United States and other countries suggest that more and more people are being diagnosed with either Crohn's disease or ulcerative colitis. One study in Finland found that the number of children with CD and UC had doubled in the last twenty years. Even in countries like India, where IBD was once unheard of, many people are being diagnosed with the condition. Therefore, IBD is no longer a rare disease, and there is evidence that it is becoming more common throughout the world.

Family History and Genetics

It has been recognized for a long time that IBD seems to run in families. About 15 to 20 percent of people with IBD have close relatives with the disease. Evidence also suggests that people with IBD who develop their illness during childhood are more likely to have other family members with IBD, compared with people whose illness begins when they are adults. A very large study of adults with IBD living in Denmark found that the children of adults with IBD had a two to thirteen times higher risk of either CD or UC than did the children of parents without IBD. In addition, people with IBD may be more likely to have family members with other autoimmune diseases, such as thyroid disease or rheumatoid arthritis.

Nonetheless, IBD is not exclusively hereditary. We know that this is true from information gathered in identical twin studies. Among identical twins, when one twin develops Crohn's disease, the likelihood of the other twin developing the same illness is about 50 percent. By contrast, if one identical twin develops ulcerative colitis, the other twin will develop UC only about 15 percent of the time. Therefore, although having an identical twin with IBD greatly increases a person's risk of developing IBD, in many twin pairs, one twin has IBD and the other doesn't.

Once it was understood that family history increases the risk of developing either CD or UC, formal genetic studies were done on families to gather more information. Geneticists are scientists who study how parental traits, or characteristics, are transmitted via genes to children. A mother and a father both transmit genes to their children, and every child is a combination of genes from both the mother and the father. The genetic material within cells that determines what characteristics a child will develop is called *deoxyribonucleic acid*, or DNA. A person's DNA acquired from mother and father will determine his height, eye color, and sex. Genes can also transmit risk of disease, which is how some diseases may run in families. In the case of CD and UC, there is no one gene or DNA piece that determines whether a child will develop these diseases. IBD is a *polygenic disease*; in other words, many genes (some from each parent) probably play a role.

IBD is also called a *complex disease*, which means both that there are many different types of IBD and that genes and environment together play a role in determining whether a person will get the disease. Environmental factors may determine if the disease will occur, when it will occur, and the types of signs and symptoms a person will show. Because IBD is a complex disease, identifying the specific genes that cause it is very difficult. In the past ten years, however, major progress has been made in studies of the heredity of IBD. In 2001, it was determined that about 25 percent of people with CD have an abnormal gene called NOD2 (otherwise known as CARD 15). More recent studies, involving large collaborations between many universities, have shown that more than 150 genes may be associated with either CD or UC.

What precisely do these genes do? Although the functions of the genes involved in IBD have yet to be resolved, current evidence suggests that these genes have at least two major roles:

1. The genes determine how the immune system cells react to intestinal bacteria. Bacteria are normally present in the intestine, but if the body's immune system sees these bacteria as invaders, or *pathogens*, inappropriate inflammation may occur.

2. The genes also determine how different cells of the immune system talk to each other (this is called *immune regulation*). Immune cells communicate with each other by chemicals

called *cytokines*, or *chemokines*. If the wrong communication is going on between cells, inappropriate inflammation may occur.

The genetics of IBD are very complex. The complexity of the genetics makes it unlikely that a genetic test for Crohn's disease or ulcerative colitis will be developed in the near future. Still, unraveling the genetics may help us better understand what causes these conditions and how best to treat them.

The Environment

The studies of genetics in IBD are challenging, but research on environmental risk factors is even more challenging. Because IBD is a rare disease, scientists need to study large numbers of people to identify environmental risk factors. In addition, an environmental risk factor may not cause (or trigger) a disease until after many years *of* exposure or until many years *after* an exposure. For example, it can take thirty years of a poor diet, smoking, and lack of exercise before a person develops diabetes or heart disease. The lapse of time between exposure and disease can make it difficult to prove the association (or link) between the environmental trigger and the onset of disease. IBD is clearly more common in the modern era, but many factors of modern life might be associated with the rise in IBD, including changes in diet, decreased physical activity, altered environmental bacteria, and decreased childhood infections. The section below summarizes the environmental risk factors that may play a role. The research in this area is inconclusive, however, and the precise environmental causes remain a topic of active study.

Diet and IBD

One of the first questions that parents ask after their child has been diagnosed with IBD is "What should my child eat?" Unfortunately, this is a very difficult question for a physician to answer. Unlike food allergies or celiac disease (a bowel disease triggered by an immunologic reaction to wheat, rye, and barley), IBD is not caused by a specific food. Some people report that certain foods may make symptoms worse, but these foods vary from person to person. A physician or nutritionist cannot prescribe a diet that will help everyone for a few reasons:

- IBD affects different individuals in diverse ways.
- Available research does not agree on the role of diet in the development of IBD.
- Good studies are difficult to perform and often require remembering details of eating habits going back several years before diagnosis.
- The patient may have altered her diet at the beginning of symptoms, before a diagnosis was confirmed.

Some studies have shown a connection between eating processed hydrogenated fats, such as margarine, and the start of CD and UC. In Japan, cases of IBD have increased with a shift to a more westernized diet lower in fish oil and higher in animal fat. Other studies have suggested that refined sugars and processed carbohydrates are associated with an increased risk of IBD, and that higher intake of fruits and vegetables reduces the risk of developing the disease. Much more research is needed.

When a child is newly diagnosed with IBD, the first instinct of the parent may be to modify the child's diet. Indeed, some children with CD will benefit from receiving a special liquid diet, called the *elemental diet*, under a physician's supervision (see chapter 13). Unfortunately, aside from the elemental diet, there is no conclusive medical evidence that making dietary changes *after* developing IBD will control the disease. Although many "special diets" that are supposed to treat IBD are available on the Internet and in the general media, these diets have not been well studied (see chapter 14). "Alternative diets" may benefit some people, but they should not be viewed as a substitute for conventional medical treatment.

Other Environmental Risk Factors

Many studies have shown that cigarette smoking is associated with a higher risk of developing Crohn's disease and may be a risk factor for flares of CD. On the other hand, in ulcerative colitis, smoking may decrease the risk of flaring up. The negative health effects of smoking far outweigh any effects smoking may have on UC flares, however, and it is strongly recommended that people with UC not smoke. Oral contraceptives may slightly increase the risk of CD in women, but most women with IBD can safely take oral contraceptives. Immunizations have not been associated with increased risk of developing IBD.

Intestinal Bacteria: An "Environmental" Cause

Trillions of bacteria live in the lumen of the human intestine (figure 2.1). They populate the intestinal fluid but are kept out of the human body by the intestinal lining (epithelium). More than four hundred different species of bacteria can be found in the large intestine, and most of these bacteria are normal inhabitants (*commensals*) of the human body. They even have beneficial functions—they help us digest food and make certain vitamins (for example, vitamin K). These normal bacteria may help

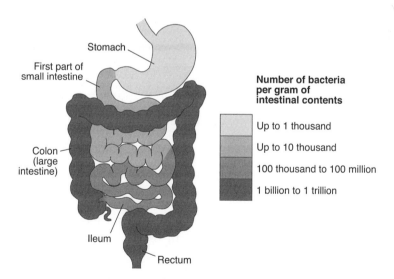

Figure 2.1. Bacteria living in the human intestine. The gastrointestinal tract is colonized by more than 100 trillion bacteria, and the numbers of bacteria increase farther down the intestine. The stomach and upper intestine have relatively few bacteria in the lumen, while the large intestine has trillions.

protect us against invasion by disease-causing (*pathogenic*) bacteria. In most people, the "normal" bacteria populating the human intestine live peacefully in our bodies and do not cause inflammation.

What's different in people with IBD? Evidence is mounting that in people with IBD, the inflammation results when the person's immune system inappropriately responds to some of these normal bacteria. Some of the evidence comes from animal models. Mice that are genetically designed to develop colitis usually do not develop colitis when grown in germ-free, sterile environments. The colitis does not occur until the intestines of these mice are colonized with "normal" bacteria. In humans, antibiotics or other antibacterial treatments may reduce the severity of IBD, possibly by reducing the number of normal bacteria in the intestines. Many studies using sophisticated DNA fingerprinting technology are currently under way to determine whether some species of normal bacteria can cause IBD in humans.

Although bacteria may play a role in triggering IBD flares, many studies have failed to conclusively demonstrate a specific bacterial or viral "cause" of IBD. Organisms that have been studied include the tuberculosis bacteria, the nontuberculous atypical mycobacteria, clostridial species, and the measles virus. Almost all these studies have been inconclusive, and most scientists believe that IBD is not caused by one species of bacteria. However, the study of the bacteria and other microorganisms in the intestine—collectively known as the intestinal *microbiome*—has become a very active area of research.

Increasing Cleanliness: The Hygiene Hypothesis

IBD, like many other immune-related diseases, may be the result of our society's improving cleanliness. (The theory involving increasing cleanliness is called the *hygiene hypothesis*.) In essence, over the past two to three decades, we have developed a wide range of products that take microbes away from our living space, from antibacterial soaps for washing dishes and laundry to antibiotics in our food sources. Thus, adults and children in countries with increasingly sterile environments are becoming more protected from routine infections (including chicken pox and *Salmonella*). Obviously, having protection from infections like chicken pox and *Salmonella* has many benefits; these infections can make people very ill and even kill some of the people they infect.

But living in an overly clean environment might have drawbacks. Exposure to normal community-acquired infections may be important for the proper development of the immune system. The hygiene hypothesis proposes that lack of regular childhood infectious exposures might have a detrimental effect on the immune system, thus increasing the risk of immune-mediated diseases like diabetes, asthma, and IBD. Following this line of thought, some scientists hypothesize that overprotection from childhood infections may lead to the wrong immune response later in life. Although this hypothesis has not been proved, the combination of better living standards, lack of exposure to gut parasites, and exposure to new environmental factors could lead to increased vulnerability to IBD. In support of this theory, we find that people growing up on farms and exposed to farm animals in early childhood may be at lower risk for developing IBD.

Does Stress Cause IBD?

Stress is not the cause of IBD, but it may make symptoms worse. Some data show that chemicals (called *neuropeptides*) released by the brain and gut during periods of stress may increase the activity of the immune system. In addition, stressful situations may make a person less likely to go to the doctor or take his medications, which can result in flares of IBD. Managing stress and anxiety may therefore be helpful in controlling IBD symptoms.

The Immune System: IBD's Pathway

Whatever causes IBD, whether one factor or many, the result is that the body's own immune system inappropriately reacts against portions of the human intestine, causing inflammation. The intestine of a person who

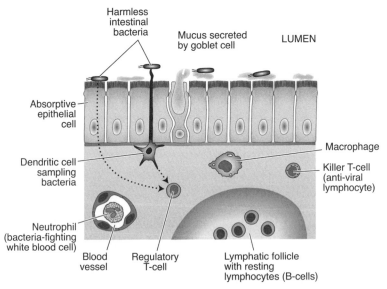

Harmless intestinal bacteria

Mucus secreted by goblet cell

LUMEN

Absorptive epithelial cell

Macrophage

Dendritic cell sampling bacteria

Killer T-cell (anti-viral lymphocyte)

Neutrophil (bacteria-fighting white blood cell)

Blood vessel

Regulatory T-cell

Lymphatic follicle with resting lymphocytes (B-cells)

Healthy intestinal lining (magnified view)

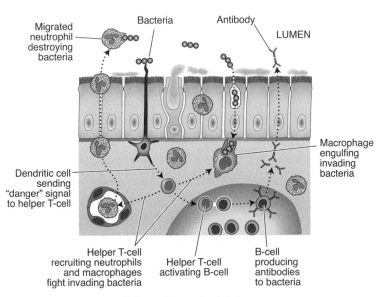

Migrated neutrophil destroying bacteria

Bacteria

Antibody

LUMEN

Dendritic cell sending "danger" signal to helper T-cell

Macrophage engulfing invading bacteria

Helper T-cell recruiting neutrophils and macrophages fight invading bacteria

Helper T-cell activating B-cell

B-cell producing antibodies to bacteria

Inflamed intestinal lining (magnified view)

has CD or UC contains too many activated immune system cells. These cells damage normal gut tissues, resulting in redness, swelling, and ulcers of the intestinal lining, and causing the person to feel pain.

Explaining all facets of how the immune system works requires a college semester and is beyond the scope of this book. For those interested, however, the section below provides a brief summary of what the immune system is and how it "goes wrong" in IBD. This understanding may be helpful later in the book because most of our currently effective treatments for IBD work by reducing the activity of the immune system.

The intestine's immune system is designed mostly to repel harmful invaders (bacteria and viruses) from the body. Such invaders (for example, *Salmonella* and *E. coli* bacteria) are very common, yet relatively few people get sick from them, because the immune system is able to repel and kill the harmful bacteria.

The major components of the immune system are the white blood cells that live in the blood, tissues, and intestinal lining. In the intestine, some white blood cells are free floating and others are clustered in what are called *lymphoid nodules*. The cells of the immune system have different functions. Some cells are "lookouts" who sense invaders and notify the rest of the body: these include epithelial cells and dendritic cells. Other cells are "soldiers" who can move in and kill bacteria and viruses by eating them or by making antibodies. The main soldiers are called B-cells, killer T-cells, and macrophages. The last group of cells are the "master control cells"; they know when to turn the immune response on and off. Master control cells, like helper T-cells, turn on the immune system when there is an infection, while other cells, called suppressor and regulatory T-cells, turn off the immune system after the infection is over (figure 2.2).

Figure 2.2. The lining of the intestine consists of cells that absorb nutrients (epithelial cells), and cells that produce intestinal mucus. Normally, bacteria are present both in the lumen and on the intestinal lining. Beneath the intestinal cell lining are several cells of the immune system that normally protect the body from infections (*top*). When the intestine is inflamed (*bottom*), more inflammatory cells (T-cells, B-cells, neutrophils) enter the intestinal wall.

Many different studies have examined what goes wrong in IBD to cause a person's immune system to react against her intestine. As with other studies of what causes IBD, there is no single conclusion. In some people, the intestinal lookouts may react improperly to intestinal bacteria. In others, soldier cells may make excessive antibodies. The master control cells may be altered in some people with IBD, and once the immune system is turned on, it may be difficult (or impossible) to turn off, resulting in uncontrolled inflammation. Knowledge gained by studying the genetics of IBD should ultimately help scientists who study the immune system to better understand these reactions.

Scientists have made tremendous progress in determining how intestinal inflammation comes about in IBD, but much more work needs to be done. Questions that have yet to be answered include the following:

1. Does any one gene or group of genes correlate with a specific type of IBD?
2. Which bacterial species, or groups of bacteria, might cause a genetically susceptible person to develop IBD?
3. Can bacterial populations in the intestine be altered through diet to decrease the risk of IBD?
4. Is there a way to reduce the activity of the immune system and control IBD without using medications that suppress the immune system?

These questions can be answered only through additional research. By participating in or funding research, parents can help doctors and scientists find the cause of IBD. We hope finding the cause may help prevent this disease in future generations.

🔲 3

Why Is IBD So Difficult to Diagnose?

If your child has already been diagnosed with either Crohn's disease or ulcerative colitis, her doctor will have already completed most of the health evaluation steps discussed in this chapter. Why, then, are we reviewing how doctors diagnose IBD? Because you may be wondering about the tests your child has had and what they find. Or you may have questions about how your doctor interprets these tests. Finally, you may be wondering, "Is the doctor right? Does my child really have IBD?"

In this chapter, we review how health care professionals evaluate a child for IBD, and which tests will prove or disprove the diagnosis. While reading this chapter, keep in mind that at diagnosis, a person with IBD must have evidence of inflammation but no evidence of an infection that would cause the inflammation. Evidence of inflammation may be seen

- at the time of physical examination
- on laboratory testing of blood or stool
- on imaging studies
- during an endoscopic examination

If a child has no evidence of inflammation on testing, the child probably does not have IBD.

Symptoms and Signs that Make a Physician Suspect IBD

Ulcerative colitis and Crohn's disease can affect different portions of the intestine. Significant inflammation in UC is usually seen only in the lower (large) intestine (colon). In contrast, CD can affect the large and small intestine. Most people with ulcerative colitis or indeterminate colitis have the symptom of bloody diarrhea. In contrast, patients with CD often have less-specific symptoms, including abdominal pain, nonbloody diarrhea, weight loss, anemia, and tiredness.

IBD can be a sneaky disease, and for some people with IBD, several months pass between the time symptoms start and the time of diagnosis. IBD can be sneaky for many reasons, with a lag time to diagnosis. Symptoms may be mild and intermittent, for example. Also, many conditions far more common than IBD cause a symptom like abdominal pain. A doctor may not consider IBD when a patient has recurrent stomachaches. Before physicians can take steps to establish the diagnosis of inflammatory bowel disease, they must first suspect that the person may have IBD.

Another reason IBD can be difficult to diagnose is that some children and teenagers are embarrassed by the symptoms and fail to tell their parents or the doctor what is really going on. Parents may be concerned about the invasiveness of tests such as colonoscopy and choose to "wait and see" before moving forward with testing. Another factor is that in a child with IBD, physical examinations and lab work are sometimes normal. In addition, some children with IBD may first see a doctor with symptoms outside the intestine, such as joint swelling, skin rashes, or eye inflammation.

Sometimes, though, IBD is anything but sneaky. Instead, it is extremely dramatic—for example, the child suddenly has severe bloody diarrhea as a symptom of UC. Bloody diarrhea is usually an alarming symptom that can frighten the child and the parent. Under these circumstances, a parent or child might ask for medical attention earlier rather than later. The doctor may need to rule out infection in the intestines before starting specific tests for IBD. (Some patients have both IBD and infection when their disease first causes symptoms.)

If the child's abdominal pain is mild and his general lifestyle and activity level are not affected, the correct diagnosis will often be delayed. Over time, as symptoms progress, it becomes easier to make the decision to start extensive testing. Table 3.1 lists some common symptoms and signs of IBD that are also seen in other diseases.

Table 3.1
Symptoms of IBD and other conditions

IBD symptom	What else might cause these symptoms?[*]
Anorexia (no appetite, refusing to eat)	• Anorexia nervosa
Weight loss, fatigue, or inability to keep up with peers	• Anemia • Malignancy (cancer) • Tuberculosis (TB)
Growth failure (not growing at a normal rate for the age) in a child with no other symptoms	• Endocrine (hormone) problems • Celiac disease
Repeated abdominal pain (stomachaches)	• Lactose intolerance • Infection with *Giardia* (a parasite) • Constipation • Functional abdominal pain • Irritable bowel syndrome (IBS)
Persistent diarrhea	• Lactose intolerance • Infection with *Giardia* • Celiac disease • Irritable bowel syndrome (IBS)
Bloody diarrhea	• Infection
Rectal bleeding	• Infection • Polyps (small growths in the colon)
Pain around the anus, with or without discharge	• Constipation • Hemorrhoids • Fissures
Constipation	• Irritable bowel syndrome (IBS)
Joint pain or swelling	• Rheumatoid arthritis • Connective tissue disease
Skin rash	• Infection • Connective tissue disease • Allergic reaction
Red eye	• Infection

[*]This list of other possible causes is not exhaustive. Other conditions can cause these symptoms, too.

Tests

A physician will suspect that a person may have IBD based on a combination of signs and symptoms. The most important initial evaluation is a thorough medical history and examination by a health care provider. The history and physical exam are described in chapter 6.

Table 3.2
Tests used in diagnosing IBD

Name of test	Type of test	Purpose
Hematocrit	Blood	Measures red blood cells; looks for anemia
Erythrocyte sedimentation rate (ESR)	Blood	Measures inflammation
C-reactive protein	Blood	Measures inflammation
Serologies (ANCA, ASCA)	Blood	Looks for antibodies sometimes seen in IBD patients
Calprotectin	Stool	Measures inflammation
Stool culture	Stool	Looks for bacteria that can cause infectious colitis or sometimes trigger IBD
C. difficile toxin	Stool	Measures protein produced by C. difficile, a bacteria that can trigger IBD flares
Upper GI and small bowel series	Radiology	Uses x-rays to evaluate the small intestine for Crohn's disease
Abdominal CT scan	Radiology	Uses x-rays to picture the intestines and the rest of the abdomen for IBD and infection
Abdominal MRI scan	Radiology	Uses magnetic imagery to picture the intestines and the rest of the abdomen for IBD and infection
Upper endoscopy	Scope	Looks for inflammation with a flexible tube inserted past the mouth and into the stomach
Colonoscopy	Scope	Looks for inflammation with a flexible tube inserted past the anus and into the large intestine
Biopsy	Microscope	Looks for microscopic signs of Crohn's disease or ulcerative colitis in small tissue samples taken during endoscopy and colonoscopy
Video capsule study	Capsule	Looks for difficult-to-find Crohn's disease in the small intestine through a small pill camera that the patient swallows and that travels down the intestine, taking hundreds of pictures

If the history and examination suggest either Crohn's disease or ulcerative colitis, additional tests will need to be performed. These tests are important for several reasons:

- to confirm the diagnosis of IBD
- to exclude other conditions that might cause similar symptoms
- to differentiate between Crohn's disease and ulcerative colitis
- to determine the severity of disease, which in turn guides treatment
- to evaluate other organ systems sometimes affected by inflammation, including the liver, skin, and eyes

Tests for IBD include blood tests, stool examinations, and radiographic imaging studies. The definitive diagnosis of IBD is usually made by directly examining the esophagus, stomach, and upper part of the intestine with an endoscope (in a test called an *upper endoscopy*), and by examining the colon and the last part of the small intestine (*ileum*) with a colonoscope (*colonoscopy*). During these tests, small samples from the intestine can be obtained for a pathologist to examine under a microscope. (Tissue taken during tests such as these is called a *biopsy*.) In patients for whom the diagnosis is strongly suspected but other tests are normal, a specialized device called a video capsule, or pill camera, may be used to take pictures of the small intestine. Table 3.2 summarizes the common tests physicians order when diagnosing and following complications of IBD. These tests are discussed in detail in part 2.

▣ Part II
Diagnosing IBD

▣ 4

The Symptoms of IBD

The symptoms of IBD are often common symptoms of any illness that affects the gastrointestinal (GI) tract. In this chapter we review some of the typical symptoms seen in children with IBD and the various causes of these symptoms. Even after a child is diagnosed, two of the most common concerns a parent has are "How do I know when my child is sick?" and "How do I know what to worry about?" Because children with IBD can develop other GI illnesses, parents and physicians may have trouble distinguishing between an IBD flare and another type of illness. As a general guideline, if the abdominal symptoms are similar to what the child had when she first became ill, they often signal a flare of the disease. If an abdominal symptom is different in location, severity, duration, or nature, then the child might have a new condition.

Abdominal Pain

Pain in the abdomen (stomach or belly area) is a first symptom of IBD in 80 percent of people with the disease. But complaints of abdominal pain in children are very common, and children with IBD can have abdominal pain for many reasons. This pain can be minor and unimportant, or it can be a sign of a serious problem.

Abdominal pain can result from a range of conditions affecting various organs. The characteristics of the pain—where it hurts, when it starts, how long it lasts, and how severe it is—are all important in helping to diagnose the cause. Any long-lasting or severe abdominal pain should be

Table 4.1
Some causes of abdominal pain in children with IBD

IBD related
- Inflammatory pain (both Crohn's disease and ulcerative colitis)
- Abdominal abscess (Crohn's disease only)
- Bowel obstruction (usually in Crohn's disease or after surgery)

May or may not be IBD related

• Gallstones	• Constipation
• Pancreatitis	• Recurrent abdominal pain of childhood (RAP)
• Appendicitis	• Irritable bowel syndrome (IBS)
• Kidney stones	• Muscle or bone pain
• Gynecological problems	• Gastroesophageal reflux (GER)
• Peptic (stomach) ulcers	• Lactose intolerance

evaluated by a doctor. Table 4.1 lists causes of abdominal pain in children with ulcerative colitis or Crohn's disease. Some of these problems are complications of the IBD itself, while others occur in children without IBD as well as in children with IBD.

Causes of Abdominal Pain Related to the Underlying IBD

Inflammatory Pain

Inflammatory pain occurs when a region of small intestine or colon is swollen, red, and sore. This type of pain can be seen in either Crohn's disease or ulcerative colitis. When the inflammation involves the colon (as in UC), pain typically occurs around the time of bowel movements and is accompanied by diarrhea or blood. In CD if the inflammation is limited to the small intestine, the child may not necessarily have pain and diarrhea with the inflammation. Inflammatory pain is a sign of a flare, or a sign that the IBD may need to be treated more aggressively. Figure 4.1 shows areas of the abdomen that may become inflamed: the colon, ileum, kidney, liver, gallbladder, or pancreas.

Abdominal Abscess

An abdominal abscess (*intra-abdominal infection*) is a complication of Crohn's disease; children with ulcerative colitis almost never get one. An abdominal

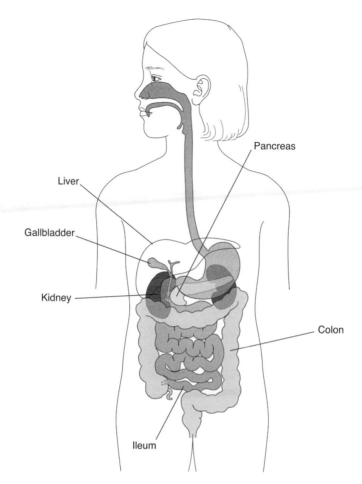

Figure 4.1. Digestive system with areas of abdomen that may become inflamed. Abdominal pain can result from inflammation of many different organs, not just the intestine. Physicians can often guess what the problem is based on the location of the pain. For example, the pancreas is located in the upper abdomen, the gallbladder is located in the right upper abdomen, and the kidneys are located in the flank.

abscess is formed when CD causes a hole (*perforation*) to develop in the bowel, usually in the small intestine (figure 4.2). When intestinal contents leak through the perforation, an infection develops. The symptoms are similar to appendicitis and include the sudden onset of significant belly pain and fever.

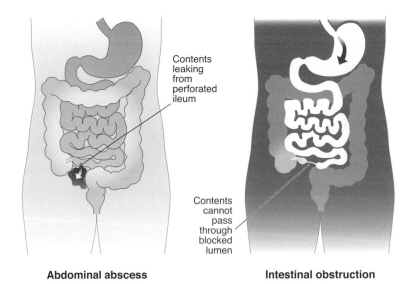

Contents
leaking
from
perforated
ileum

Contents
cannot
pass
through
blocked
lumen

Abdominal abscess   **Intestinal obstruction**

Figure 4.2. Abdominal abscess and intestinal obstruction. These two complications of Crohn's disease usually result from inflammation in the small
intestine. In an abdominal abscess, a hole in the intestine (usually in the
ileum) results in the leakage of fluid into the abdomen, mimicking what is
seen in a perforated appendix. In an intestinal obstruction (stricture), an area
of the intestine becomes scarred, so that contents have trouble passing.

Bowel Obstruction

A bowel obstruction means that food and fluid are having trouble moving
through the bowel because of a mechanical blockage. In CD (but not in
UC), obstructions may develop if the small intestine scars internally and
becomes narrow. Another cause of a bowel obstruction is *adhesions* (kinks
in the bowel that may occur after surgery). Children with obstructions
typically have a sudden onset of severe belly pain and vomiting, and the
symptoms should be treated as an emergency. A careful physical examination and an abdominal x-ray will make it possible to diagnose most obstructions (see figure 4.2).

Causes of Abdominal Pain that May, or May Not, Be Related to IBD

Gallstones

Gallstones are seldom a cause of abdominal pain in children and teens. The gallbladder is a small sac located next to the liver that helps store digestive juices. Small stones can form inside the sac and irritate the gallbladder or the tubes that drain the liver, causing pain. Gallstones can also cause inflammation of the pancreas (see pancreatitis, below) if the stone blocks the flow of digestive juices out of the pancreas. Gallbladder pain can be either sharp or dull and is usually felt on the right side of the abdomen, under the ribcage. Pain from the gallbladder usually starts a few minutes after a meal, especially if the meal is high in fat. Most gallstones can be easily detected by an ultrasound. If recurrent abdominal pain is the result of gallstones, the gallstones and gallbladder should be removed. Children with IBD may have an increased risk of developing gallstones.

Pancreatitis

Pancreatitis is inflammation of a digestive organ called the pancreas, which is in the middle of the abdomen. The inflammation causes an injury to the pancreas. In children, pancreatitis may occur without explanation, but it can also be caused by gallstones, infections, and medications. Some of the medicines used to treat IBD, such as azathioprine, 6-mercaptopurine, and 5-aminosalicylates, can cause pancreatitis. Children with CD can also develop pancreatitis as a result of inflammation of their small intestine.

Children with pancreatitis typically have a sudden onset of abdominal pain, back pain, or vomiting. People with IBD say that the pain from pancreatitis is "different" from the pain of a flare. The diagnosis of pancreatitis can usually be easily established with a blood test; an ultrasound or CT scan is often done to exclude gallstones. The symptoms of pancreatitis usually improve after a few hours or days of decreased eating as well as hydration with intravenous fluids. If it is suspected that a medication is causing the pancreatitis, then the medication will probably need to be discontinued.

Appendicitis

Appendicitis is the most common condition requiring emergency abdominal surgery in children, but it can occur at any age. Appendicitis happens when the inside of the appendix is blocked, leading to reduced blood flow away from the area. Classic symptoms of appendicitis include fever, nausea, vomiting, and pain. It can be difficult to distinguish appendicitis from a flare in children with CD, although appendicitis usually has a more sudden onset than a flare. Tests such as ultrasound and CT scans are helpful. The treatment of acute appendicitis is surgery to remove the appendix. Surgery usually happens within several hours after confirming the diagnosis.

Kidney Stones

Kidney stones can occur in anyone, but they are more common in people with CD. The symptoms of kidney stones include back and side pain, vomiting, and blood in the urine. The stones usually can easily be seen with an ultrasound. The standard treatment is intravenous fluid and pain medication.

Gynecological Problems

Gynecological problems (problems involving the female reproductive organs) can cause abdominal pain in teenage girls. These problems include pelvic infections or inflammation, sexually transmitted infections, abnormal periods, pregnancy, or diseases of the ovaries. The pain can be located in the middle of the abdomen, or only in the lower right or left side; if the pain is in the lower abdomen, it may resemble IBD pain. Cysts on the ovaries can cause lower abdominal pain halfway through a girl's cycle. Tests for gynecological problems include urinalysis (checking the urine), urine culture, pregnancy testing, a pelvic exam, and screening for infections.

Peptic (Stomach and Duodenal) Ulcers

Ulcers are wounds that can occur in the stomach or lining of the intestine. In healthy people, they most commonly occur in the stomach or in the first part of the small intestine. Ulcers occur in people with Crohn's disease and in people with ulcerative colitis, though they occur more often in people with CD. If a person with IBD has been taking aspirin, nonsteroidal anti-inflammatory drugs (NSAIDs) such as ibuprofen, or steroids for a long time, then medication may be the cause of an ulcer. The most common symptoms of an ulcer are pain and bleeding.

Constipation

Constipation is one of the most common reasons that children visit the pediatrician's office because of abdominal pain. While IBD most often causes diarrhea, some patients with IBD may also have constipation. Constipation can sometimes cause severe pain—it can feel like, or be mistaken for, appendicitis. Diagnosis of constipation is done by taking a careful history, performing a physical examination (which might include a rectal exam), and sometimes ordering an abdominal x-ray. Treatment of constipation in children usually involves giving them stool softeners or laxatives and educating the child and family on how to avoid stool-holding behaviors.

Recurrent Abdominal Pain

Recurrent abdominal pain (RAP) of childhood is a condition in which a child has repeated bouts of abdominal pain without an obvious physical explanation. By definition, children with RAP have at least three episodes of abdominal pain over at least three months. This definition applies to children who are 3 years or older. The pain is usually severe enough to get in the way of daily activities, but it does not have a clear cause. RAP affects nearly 1 out of 10 school-age children. More girls than boys are affected by RAP. The pain usually occurs only around the belly button area and is usually vague (not easy to localize); a short rest can be enough to relieve the pain. Treatment with antacids or pain relievers does not usually help.

Doctors think that about 25 percent of children with RAP may grow up to have irritable bowel syndrome.

Irritable Bowel Syndrome

Irritable bowel syndrome (IBS) is one of the most common conditions affecting the bowel, affecting an estimated 15 percent of people in the United States. IBS is also known as spastic colon. Some doctors may call IBS "colitis" (inflammation of the large intestine), but the term is inaccurate here, because there is no inflammation. Symptoms of IBS include looser and more frequent bowel movements, straining while passing stool, urgency, and bloating. Distinguishing between IBS and IBD requires knowing all medical history of the patient, as well as using laboratory tests. If there is no anemia (low red blood cell count) and no signs of inflammation in special blood tests, the problem is probably IBS. In children who have IBD, however, colonoscopy may be needed to distinguish between an IBD flare and IBS.

Muscle or Bone Pain

Muscle or bone pain is not unusual after exercise. It can be difficult to tell the difference between exercise-related pain and more serious causes of abdominal pain. In exercise-related pain, there should be no trouble with bowel movements, no vomiting or fever, and the pain should get better after taking simple pain relievers such as acetaminophen or ibuprofen.

Gastroesophageal Reflux

Gastroesophageal reflux (GER) can cause abdominal pain, usually in the middle of the upper abdomen and spreading up into the chest. There may be nausea or a feeling of food coming up into the esophagus (food pipe) and mouth. The pain often starts 30 minutes to 1 hour after a meal, especially a large meal, but it can occur at any time. Specific foods, such as carbonated drinks, caffeine, and tomato products, can make GER worse. Antacids can help decrease discomfort. Patients with IBD may also have symptoms of GER, especially if the IBD affects the stomach or esophagus.

Lactose Intolerance

Lactose intolerance can cause abdominal pain with increased intestinal gas and diarrhea. Lactose, or milk sugar, is found in dairy products and in most baked goods. About 20 percent of Caucasian adults, and up to 80 percent of African Americans and Asian Americans, have lactose intolerance. People with IBD, particularly older children and young adults, may also have lactose intolerance. When people who are lactose intolerant eat products containing lactose, they develop symptoms of pain, gas, diarrhea, and bloating, usually 30 to 60 minutes after ingestion. Treatment of lactose intolerance involves cutting back on milk products and taking pills that contain lactase enzyme, which can be bought at pharmacies or grocery stores. Lactose intolerance is not an allergy to milk, and many lactose-intolerant individuals can tolerate small to moderate amounts of milk or cheese.

Diarrhea

As with abdominal pain, diarrhea is a symptom of multiple possible illnesses. In this section, we describe the clues that help distinguish between IBD and another cause of diarrhea.

Many conditions can cause diarrhea (table 4.2). Some of these conditions may feel like flares of CD or UC. If the cause of the diarrhea is unclear, your child's doctor can examine him and order laboratory tests. The physical exam and laboratory tests can usually determine the cause of the symptoms—whether it is IBD or something else.

Bloody Diarrhea

Bloody diarrhea with cramps is one of the most common symptoms of IBD. Very often, in a child who has been diagnosed with UC or CD, the physician will simply treat for an IBD flare. Even so, it is important always to consider infection as a cause of the diarrhea, especially if the episode starts suddenly. Several common bacterial infections can cause bloody diarrhea, including *Salmonella*, *Shigella*, *Campylobacter*, *Yersinia*, and

Table 4.2
Causes of diarrhea in children with IBD

Bloody diarrhea	Nonbloody diarrhea
• Flare of IBD	• Irritable bowel syndrome
• Acute bacterial infections:	• Lactose intolerance
Salmonella	• Diarrhea after bowel surgery, due to
Shigella	rapid transit (food moving too fast
Campylobacter	through the intestines)
Yersinia	too much bile acid in the colon
Escherichia coli	malabsorption (inability of the small
• Clostridium difficile infection	intestine to absorb important
• Amoeba infection (in people who	vitamins and other nutrients from
recently traveled to areas of the world	food)
where this organism is common)	bacterial overgrowth (too many
	bacteria in the intestines)
	• Prescribed medications
	• Herbs and dietary supplements
	• Too much juice or sugarless gum
	• Celiac disease
	• Excessive laxatives

E. coli. These infections usually occur when a person eats contaminated food. Especially risky are undercooked chicken (which can contain *Salmonella* and *Campylobacter*) and undercooked ground beef (which can contain *E. coli*).

Another bacterium that can cause bloody diarrhea is *Clostridium difficile* (also referred to as *C. difficile* or *C. diff*). This infection often occurs when a person has recently received antibiotics or has recently been hospitalized, but more recently it is being acquired in the community setting. *C. difficile* infection is common in people with IBD and can recur after treatment is stopped. When people travel abroad, bloody diarrhea can also be caused by organisms not commonly seen in the United States, such as amoeba. Thus, it is important to inform your doctor if your family has traveled abroad recently.

Treatment is determined by which infection is causing the diarrhea. The cause of bacterial and amoebic colitis can usually be identified by a single stool culture, though multiple stool cultures may be necessary. A stool culture means checking to see if known disease-causing organisms (for example, bacteria) grow in the stool. Special tests are needed to identify *C. difficile* and amoebic colitis. Unlike IBD colitis, most cases of bacterial colitis usually disappear on their own or get better with antibiotic treatment. In people with IBD, bleeding from the anus that lasts more than two weeks with negative cultures is probably due to an IBD flare.

Nonbloody Diarrhea

Nonbloody diarrhea is very common in the general population and has many different causes. Most people with ulcerative colitis usually have bleeding in addition to diarrhea when their disease flares. On the other hand, people with Crohn's disease (particularly CD in the small intestine) can have nonbloody diarrhea, especially if they have had bowel surgery.

Acute nonbloody diarrhea (a sudden attack of mushy or watery diarrhea) is usually caused by a virus. Viruses generally affect the lining of the small intestine, causing oozing of intestinal fluid. Viruses also limit the absorption (taking in) of food from the small intestine. Viral infections of the intestines often spread from person to person, mainly through saliva or infected stools. For example, viral infection of the intestines spreads rapidly among young children in daycare settings. Nausea, vomiting, and low-grade fevers (usually 101° or less) are normal in children with viral illnesses. Diarrhea from a viral infection usually lasts between three to seven days, though some illnesses can last as long as fourteen days. A stool sample test can identify some of these viruses but not others. However, since most viral infections are self-limited, and antibiotic treatment is not indicated, doctors typically do not recommend viral stool tests.

In people without IBD, chronic nonbloody diarrhea can commonly be caused by either IBS or lactose intolerance (see previous section on abdominal pain). The results of diagnostic tests, including blood tests, stool cultures, and colonoscopy (see chapters 7–9), are normal in people with IBS. These normal tests help distinguish IBS from the different forms of IBD. To complicate things somewhat, however, patients with IBD (either Crohn's disease or ulcerative colitis) can also have IBS. In some cases, the best way to tell the difference between symptoms arising from IBS and those from a mild flare of IBD is with a colonoscopy. If the colonoscopy and biopsies suggest that the IBD is under control, then IBS should be treated.

Chronic diarrhea can occur in patients who have had bowel surgery for Crohn's disease. This is true especially if the last part of the small intestine (terminal ileum) and the first part of the large intestine (cecum) were surgically removed. The diarrhea occurs in part because things move through the shorter intestine more quickly, and in part because bile acids (digestive chemicals in the intestine) may irritate the colon. In any person with CD who has had this surgery and develops chronic non-bloody diarrhea, the first step is to make sure that the disease is not flaring. If a flare is ruled out, then diarrhea after surgery can be treated with the medication cholestyramine to reduce the bile acids. Additional helpful medications are loperamide, to slow down the movement of food through the intestines, and antibiotics such as metronidazole or ciprofloxacin, to reduce the load of some bacteria in the intestines.

When the intestines are not able to take in everything the body needs from the food the person eats, this is called *malabsorption*. Malabsorption can occur if there is widespread CD of the small intestine, or if major surgery was done on the small intestine. Malabsorption may require a modified diet and vitamin supplements.

Other causes of diarrhea do not commonly affect children with IBD. Some prescription medications for IBD, such as 5-ASA, may cause diarrhea. In addition, over-the-counter treatments such as herbal and dietary supplements may cause diarrhea. Too much juice and sugarless gum can result in a mushy or watery diarrhea. Celiac disease, a form of intolerance to wheat, can cause diarrhea, abdominal pain, and gas; the diagnosis can be established by a simple blood test and an upper endoscopy. Finally, some people with IBD may at times feel constipated; if they take too many laxatives, they may develop diarrhea.

Slowed Growth and Late Puberty

Many chronic inflammatory diseases can cause slowed growth and delayed puberty (growth failure). This is particularly true in children with IBD. Approximately 50 percent of children with Crohn's disease and 10 percent of children with ulcerative colitis will develop such symptoms. Slowed growth and delayed puberty may be the first sign of CD.

A child with IBD who is smaller and skinnier than his classmates, or whose predicted height is smaller than what his parents would expect based on their own heights, should be evaluated for growth failure. The reasons for growth failure in children with IBD are summarized in table 4.3. Fundamentally, chronic inflammation suppresses appetite, leading to decreased calories being eaten, which in turn causes undernutrition. Because the child is getting fewer calories than desired, his growth slows. Proteins involved in the inflammatory process itself (*cytokines*) and prolonged use of steroids can also result in growth failure through a direct effect on the bones. Treatment of growth failure is discussed in chapter 13.

Table 4.3
Causes of slow growth and late puberty in children with IBD

- Poor intake resulting in too few calories, caused by

    abdominal pain

    decreased appetite

    fear of eating

    nutrient deficiencies

- Inflammation's effects on puberty: direct suppression of puberty by inflammatory chemicals (cytokines)

- Poor absorption of food and calories, caused by

    loss of intestine from surgery

    decreased nutrient absorption because of intestinal inflammation

    specific vitamin deficiencies

- Prolonged use of corticosteroids to treat IBD

Liver Problems

About 5 percent of people with IBD have inflammation of the liver. The liver is a triangular organ that is located in the upper right portion of the abdomen. This organ is essential in digesting foods, making proteins, and ridding the body of toxins. Symptoms of liver disease include chronic fa-

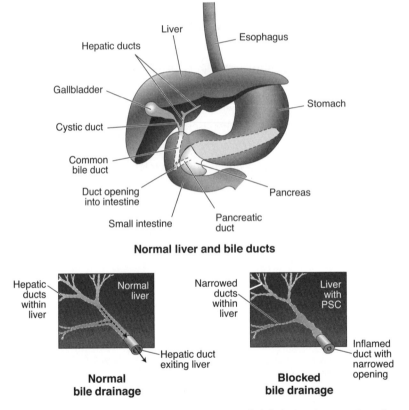

Normal liver and bile ducts

Normal bile drainage

Blocked bile drainage

Figure 4.3. The liver produces digestive juices (bile) that enter a series of small tubes called hepatic ducts and bile ducts. The digestive juices then enter the upper part of the intestine (duodenum). In a rare condition called primary sclerosing cholangitis (PSC), which a few people with IBD develop, the ducts draining the liver become narrowed and scarred.

tigue, jaundice (a yellow color to the skin), and severe itching. Your child's doctor will probably order blood tests to check liver function at least once a year. The digestive juices made in the liver leave the liver and enter the intestine through a series of tubes called *bile ducts* (figure 4.3). Primary sclerosing cholangitis (PSC) is an inflammatory disorder of the bile ducts that can cause scarring and blockages within the ducts; it occurs more commonly in UC than in CD, but it can also occur in CD. For many patients, PSC is a mild condition that can be treated with medication. Over time, though, some patients with PSC develop liver cirrhosis (scarring of the liver).

Autoimmune hepatitis (AIH) is another liver disorder that some people with IBD develop. In AIH, the body's immune system attacks the liver cells, similar to how it attacks the intestine in IBD. Most people with CD and AIH have no symptoms of hepatitis, and although the liver tests your child has every year will also screen for AIH, only a liver biopsy can confirm the diagnosis of autoimmune hepatitis. Drug treatment of AIH with the medications prednisone and azathioprine usually controls the disease.

People with IBD, especially CD, are prone to develop gallstones (*cholelithiasis*). The risk increases if they are not allowed to take in food or drinks by mouth for a length of time, for example, if they get nutrition through a vein (known as *parenteral nutrition*), or if they require treatment with corticosteroids.

Pancreas Problems

Pancreatitis (inflammation of the pancreas) can develop in people with IBD for several reasons (see earlier section on abdominal pain). The most common is a reaction to medications that are frequently used to treat IBD. Medications known to trigger pancreatitis include sulfasalazine, mesalamine, azathioprine, and 6-mercaptopurine. In pancreatitis, the inflamed pancreas causes severe abdominal pain and vomiting. The diagnosis is easily made by the identification of elevated pancreatic proteins (amylase and lipase) in a blood test.

A typical episode of pancreatitis lasts three to five days. To treat pancreatitis, the patient is not given any food by mouth, so that the pancreas can rest. During this time the patient will receive nutrition through an IV. Rarely, pancreatitis can be severe. If a medication is believed to cause the pancreatitis, then the patient will be asked to stop taking it. Gallstones or Crohn's disease of the duodenum (part of the small intestine) can block the pancreatic duct, also causing pancreatitis. Because the pain of pancreatitis can feel like the pain of severe IBD, a careful physical and diagnostic examination is required to determine the true source of the symptoms when pancreatitis is suspected.

Symptoms from Organs Outside the Gastrointestinal Tract

Joint Pain and Inflammation

Joint pain (*arthralgia*) and joint inflammation (*arthritis*) are the most common IBD symptoms that occur outside the intestines. The knees, hips, and ankles are the joints most likely to suffer (figure 4.4). Joint pain and joint inflammation tend to occur at the same time as inflammation in the intestines. In some cases, however, joint problems may show up before the diarrhea and abdominal pain connected with IBD. The joints may ache and be painful without any obvious change in how they look. When serious inflammation is present, the joint will appear swollen, warm to the touch, or red. There may also be pain when the joint is used or examined. Very often, joint disease improves when the IBD is controlled. When the joint inflammation does not respond to treatment of the IBD, the child may benefit from consulting a pediatric rheumatologist (arthritis specialist).

Eye Problems

The eye becomes inflamed in a small percentage of children with IBD. In *episcleritis*, the most common eye problem, the *sclera* (white of the eye) and the *conjunctiva* (the inside of the eyelid and the covering in front of the eyeball) become reddened and inflamed. There is no pain or change in eyesight. This condition may look like pink eye. In *uveitis*, inflammation of the *uvea* (the middle part of the eye) causes significant pain, and the vision can become blurry and sensitive to light.

Both conditions, and particularly uveitis, require treatment by an ophthalmologist (eye doctor). The seriousness of the eye problem is not always related to the seriousness of the IBD. While eye problems are uncommon in children with IBD, your child should visit an ophthalmologist (eye doctor) regularly to identify any eye problems as early as possible.

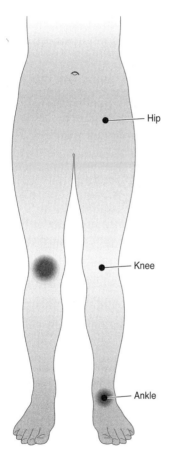

Figure 4.4. People with IBD may develop joint pain or swelling. Usually, large joints (hip, knee, ankle) are affected. In addition, the joint swelling is usually asymmetric (affecting one joint but not the same joint on the opposite side).

Your child's gastroenterologist can help you determine how often eye exams should be scheduled for your child.

Kidney Problems

Kidney stones may develop in people with IBD, particularly after surgery that involves the ileum, the last section of the small intestine. The passage of a kidney stone from the kidney into the *ureter* (the tube that carries urine to the bladder) is very painful. Kidney stones are usually diagnosed with ultrasound. Although many stones pass normally during urination, after the person receives hydration treatment, kidney stones may need to be removed surgically. Alternatively, a technique called *lithotripsy* (sound waves that break stones into smaller pieces so that they can pass normally through the ureter) may be used.

Other, rarer kidney problems that may occur in CD (but not in UC) include blockage of the ureter by an inflammatory growth, *fistulas* (abnormal openings) between the intestines and the bladder, and inflammation of the kidneys.

Skin Problems

People with IBD may develop skin rashes, some of which are associated with inflammation. *Erythema nodosum* is a rash of painful red bumps, typically on the shins, that appears in children with new onset or flaring IBD. Sometimes swelling of the feet or legs may be associated. A more severe rash, *pyoderma gangrenosum*, causes large ulcers but is very rarely seen in children. Some medications (for example, sulfasalazine) may increase sensitivity to sunlight, which makes the child more likely to get sunburned. Children with IBD may also develop allergic reactions to their medications, which look like "drug rashes."

Children with ulcerative colitis or Crohn's disease can experience many different symptoms. In some children, warning signs of a flare are obvious. In others, warning signs may be subtle. In addition, some children may visit the doctor because they think they have a flare, only to be diagnosed with some other illness. Because this happens so often, it's not a good idea to assume that every GI symptom is a flare of IBD. Both patients and physicians need to consider other diagnoses, and additional testing should be performed if needed to make a diagnosis. It is crucial for children with UC who are having new diarrhea to have stool cultures performed to rule out infections.

回 5

How to Prepare for a Visit to Your Child's IBD Doctor

Caring for a child with IBD involves a partnership between the parent and the physician. The parent and the physician work together to keep the child's IBD under control. The parent's role is to provide accurate information, ask questions, gain knowledge, and provide input into decisions about the child's treatment. The physician's responsibility is to provide accurate information, ask questions, examine the patient, assess disease severity, and recommend a treatment plan. Physicians and parents need to discuss alternatives and make choices together.

Most children with IBD in North America are cared for by pediatric gastroenterologists. A pediatric gastroenterologist is a doctor who specializes in the diagnosis and management of diseases of the digestive system in people up to age 16, 18, or sometimes 21 years. A good resource to find a pediatric gastroenterologist is the Web site of the North American Society for Pediatric Gastroenterology, Hepatology and Nutrition: www.naspghan.org. If you are reading this book, then most likely you have already consulted with a pediatric gastroenterologist. At what age a child starts seeing an adult gastroenterologist depends on the geographic location or institution where the patient is being seen. Older children and teens may be cared for by a gastroenterologist who treats mostly adult patients, although it is recommended that a pediatric gastroenterologist, if one is available, be involved in the care of any child with IBD.

Preparing for a First Visit to the Gastroenterologist

Seeing a new doctor for the first time can be exciting, especially if there is hope that the doctor will have new or helpful ideas to improve the child's health or well-being. But this visit can also be an unsettling time for parents and children, especially if they are changing from one medical practice to another or have moved to a new city or town. Some families may be reading this book while in the process of changing from an adult to a pediatric gastroenterologist (or vice versa), changing from one pediatric gastroenterologist to another, or moving from one town to another. Many families are happy with their current care but want to obtain another opinion about medical treatment. Whether for a first visit to a new doctor or a return visit, a parent can do much to help make the most of each appointment, and to help the doctor as well. Careful preparation is the key.

The parent who arrives prepared makes it much more likely that three important goals can be reached during that first critical visit with the doctor:

1. Your gastroenterologist (and gastroenterology nurse practitioner, where applicable) will have in hand all the important medical history and test results and therefore will be better prepared to determine how to manage your child's IBD.
2. Your child will know what to expect during the visit, which will help her cooperate with the medical team.
3. Your key concerns and questions will be addressed.

How can you and your child prepare for the doctor's visit so that you can achieve the three goals listed above? Gather a history of your child's illness, get copies of medical records, and write down your questions and concerns.

Step 1. Assemble a complete history of your child's illness as well as relevant family illnesses. Try to make these histories as complete as possible.

A. Review in your own mind your child's current illness and describe it in writing.

- When did it begin?
- How often do the symptoms occur?
- How has your child been functioning: energy level, appetite, school performance, sleep?
- Have you been aware of any fevers?
- Do you think your child has lost weight or is not growing in height as expected?

B. Sit down with your child in a quiet place, away from distractions, and compare notes about when her problems and symptoms started, and how things are going now. Be prepared to discuss these topics with your child:

- Pain

    When does it happen?

    Where is it located?

    How severe is it?

    How long does it last?

    What brings it on or relieves it?

- Weight changes
- Energy level
- Sleep
- Appetite
- School performance (Has it changed because of physical discomfort?)
- Aching joints
- Fevers
- Mouth sores
- Bowel movements (stools). This is often the most difficult subject for your child to talk about:

    How many a day?

    What do they look like (including any visible blood or mucus)?

    Are they painful?

    Do they occur at night?

    Are there any sores around your child's bottom?

It can be very helpful to the physician for you to inspect your child's bowel movements a couple of times before the first visit.

C. Keep a diary of symptoms, including stools (detailed as above), for one to two weeks before the visit.

D. Make a list of all your child's medications and doses (bring this list to the doctor). Be sure to include vitamin supplements, herbal products, and any nutritional supplements your child is taking. (You could also bring all the pill containers to the visit so that the doctor can read the labels, if desired.)

E. Think about your child's medical history. Has your child ever been hospitalized or had surgery? Is he allergic to any medications or foods?

F. Contact your relatives—grandparents, aunts, uncles, first cousins of your child—and ask about a history of any of the following:
- Inflammatory bowel disease (Crohn's disease, ulcerative colitis)
- Primary sclerosing cholangitis (a liver disease affecting the bile ducts, which may cause yellowing of the skin and eyes)
- Irritable bowel syndrome (spastic colon)
- Lactose intolerance

Step 2. Obtain copies of essential medical records and test results.

A. General health information from the primary care doctor or nurse practitioner that will be helpful to the GI team includes
- childhood illnesses
- growth chart
- immunization records

B. Results from previous blood tests, which may include
- complete blood count (CBC)
- protein level (albumin)
- markers of inflammation—ESR (erythrocyte sedimentation rate), CRP (C-reactive protein)
- liver function tests (AST, ALT, bilirubin levels, alkaline phosphatase)

C. Results from stool tests, which may include

- stool culture
- *Clostridium difficile* (*C. diff* toxin)
- ova and parasites (O&P)
- *Giardia*
- calprotectin

D. Results from imaging studies, which may include
  - plain abdominal films (acute abdominal series; kidneys, ureters, and bladder, also called KUB)
  - upper gastrointestinal series (UGI) with small bowel series (also called UGI with small bowel follow-through)
  - abdominal CT (CAT) scan
  - magnetic resonance imaging (MRI)

  Bring copies of the actual films, if possible, as well as the radiologist's official report. Your primary care doctor will generally not have a copy of the actual films; you can get a copy from the laboratory or hospital where the x-rays were done.

E. Records of procedures, which may include
  - upper endoscopy (EGD)
  - colonoscopy
  - sigmoidoscopy

  When you visit the doctor, bring any pictures taken during the procedure, as well as a copy of the *endoscopist's report.* If biopsies were taken during the endoscopy, bring a copy of the *biopsy report.* Most pediatric gastroenterologists will want to review the actual biopsy slides. The GI specialist who performed the endoscopy will not have the slides. You should request them from the pathology department at the center where the procedures were performed. That department may wish to mail the slides directly to the pediatric gastroenterologist or to the pathology department in the hospital where the gastroenterologist works.

F. If your child has had any surgeries related to her digestive tract problems, bring copies of the operative report and the pathology report and slides (see discussion on procedures above).

G. Just prior to the visit, collect a stool sample from your child to bring with you to the visit. One convenient method is to collect the stool directly into a gallon-size food-storage bag and double-bag it.

Step 3. Write down a list of all the immediate concerns and any questions you and your child have. Bring this list with you to the first visit. If you don't bring a list, it's far too easy to forget your questions once the visit starts.

Preparing for Follow-Up Visits to the Gastroenterologist

Preparation always helps things go more smoothly and aids treatment decisions. Be sure to prepare for subsequent visits to the doctor, too. Ask your child to keep a diary of his symptoms, starting one to two weeks before the next scheduled follow-up visit. This diary should include everything from Step 1 above. Ask your child to include the same level of detail about these symptoms as you did for the initial visit.

Bring a list of all current medications, vitamins, and herbal supplements to the follow-up visit. Be prepared to discuss how and when your child is taking the medicines. If your child has any difficulties with taking any medicines, be honest with the doctor about this issue. Make notes beforehand of any side effects you or your child is noticing. For example, some medications can cause a rash, headaches, moodiness, or a puffy face.

Once again, write down all your questions and concerns before the visit. Bring the list with you.

Your gastroenterology health care team recognizes and appreciates the time and effort involved in thoroughly preparing for visits to their office. Your efforts will greatly enhance their ability to provide the best custom care for your child.

Helpful Dos and Don'ts for Any Visit

With the best of intentions, parents sometimes do things (or don't do things) that make the visit to the doctor more stressful for their child. Bear the following points in mind:

- Please do not promise your child that there will be no blood tests.
- Please do not look distressed when a rectal exam is done. A rectal exam involves looking at your child's bottom and sometimes probing inside with a gloved finger. This exam is often the best way to determine whether a child is in a flare. Although a rectal examination is not necessarily performed at every visit, it is sometimes needed for the doctor or nurse to provide the best care.
- Please do not look surprised when a doctor or nurse asks a child who is 13 or older to report the names and amounts of each medication he is taking. This is often the first step in helping him gain more independence and take charge of his IBD.
- Unless otherwise instructed by the office of the pediatric gastroenterologist, please *do* let your child eat prior to the visit. Procedures are seldom performed on the day of the first visit or on a follow-up visit unless a plan that includes procedures is discussed beforehand with the parent.

6

Office Visits and Procedures
for Children with IBD

Diagnosing IBD in a child, whether it is Crohn's disease or ulcerative colitis, generally involves a series of steps. The diagnosis will proceed from the basic medical interview and physical examination to simple stool tests and blood tests, as well as, when necessary, radiologic imaging studies and endoscopic tests (see chapter 9) requiring sedation or anesthesia. Only when doctors strongly suspect that a child has IBD will they suggest invasive tests, such as a colonoscopy. Severely ill children may have to enter the hospital so that doctors can run tests more quickly and so that the children can be supported better during testing.

The Medical History Interview

The first step in making the diagnosis of IBD is the medical interview of the patient and family. Doctors ask whether the child has typical symptoms (diarrhea, rectal bleeding, and abdominal cramping). They then try to assess the severity of the symptoms, how long they have been present, and whether they are getting worse. To do this, doctors obviously have to ask questions about body functions that are usually private. Although discussing bowel movements may be embarrassing for your child, these questions are extremely important.

Doctors also ask questions to find out how the disease has affected the child's overall health. For example, has your child had fever, a low energy level, weight loss, or delays in growth or puberty? Another critical part of the interview reviews other organs in the body, to assess whether extraintestinal symptoms (IBD symptoms that appear outside the digestive tract) are present.

The doctors' job is not only to assess whether a child's symptoms agree with the diagnosis of IBD, but also to reject the diagnoses of other disorders that can have similar symptoms (see chapters 3 and 4). The interview also includes a review of medical history, such as previous surgeries or hospitalizations, family history (illness that may run in the family), and social history (where and with whom the child lives, school attendance, etc.). The medical history helps doctors find out whether a child has other medical problems that might affect the diagnosis or treatment of colitis. Reviewing the family history is crucial, because as many as 20 percent of children with inflammatory bowel disease have close relatives with the disease. The social history is important to help doctors understand how the disease is affecting school attendance and other activities.

The Physical Examination

The next step in the evaluation is a complete physical examination. This usually starts with measurement of height and weight so that the child's growth and nutritional status can be assessed. Doctors examine the child's skin, checking for paleness that might suggest anemia (low level of red blood cells). They also check the skin for rashes that may accompany IBD.

The oral examination is an important component of the physical exam. Doctors look for mouth sores, which can be found in people with IBD, especially with CD. They listen to the heart and lungs. The abdomen is carefully examined for tenderness, swelling, enlargement of internal organs (such as the liver and spleen), and the presence of masses that might indicate areas of inflamed bowel.

Doctors check the anal area for other causes of bleeding, such as hemorrhoids or *fissures* (cracks in the skin), and for lesions typical of CD. A rectal examination (which requires the doctor to gently insert a gloved finger into the anus) may reveal a polyp or other abnormalities. During the rectal exam, a small stool sample may be obtained so that the laboratory can test for the presence of blood. The child's joints are examined for evidence of redness, pain, or swelling. Examination of the genitals to determine the stage of sexual maturity is important, since children with IBD often enter puberty late.

Laboratory Tests

If the history and physical examination suggest that the child may have IBD, laboratory tests are done. (Laboratory tests are often called *studies*.) Blood tests can help look for evidence of blood loss, inflammation, or nutritional deficiencies, and stool tests can identify infection. Additional blood tests can check how well other organs, such as the kidneys and liver, are working. A urinalysis (urine test) is also helpful to check kidney function. These tests are described in more detail in chapter 7.

Imaging Studies

Radiographic studies can be important in the diagnosis of IBD. Plain x-rays of the abdomen can provide general information regarding the health of the intestine and can assess whether a complication, such as a blockage or perforation (hole), has occurred. X-ray studies that use contrast liquid (either swallowed or administered rectally) can give a "big picture" view of the anatomy of the intestines. These tests are described in more detail in chapter 8.

Endoscopic Evaluation

The most valuable studies to help make the diagnosis of IBD are endoscopic procedures that use long steerable tubes with a video chip on their end. The video component allows doctors to examine the appearance of the internal lining of the upper and lower intestinal tracts. Doctors can also perform biopsies during these procedures. Biopsies involve taking small "pinch" samples of the lining of the intestine for later examination under a microscope. These tests are described in more detail in chapter 9.

What Happens after My Child Has Been Diagnosed with IBD?

IBD is a chronic and unpredictable disease characterized by periods of disease remission interspersed with disease relapses. It is usually difficult to predict when a relapse might occur. Fortunately, most children respond well to treatment and can carry on with a normal lifestyle. All children with IBD need long-term follow-up by a gastroenterology team for medical treatment, monitoring of medication side effects, treating disease complications, and most important, emotional support in the face of living with a chronic disease. In smaller practices, the team may be composed of a doctor and a nurse. In larger centers, the team may involve different doctors (gastroenterologist, endocrinologist), nurses, social workers, counselors, and a nutritionist.

How Do I Help My Family Deal with Stress during This Time?

The diagnosis of IBD may be difficult for both the child and the family. Having blood drawn, drinking contrast liquid (barium for an imaging study), and preparing for, and having, an endoscopic procedure can certainly be stressful, especially for young children.

For parents, not knowing the cause of their child's symptoms, and experiencing the fear surrounding a chronic or life-threatening illness, may be overwhelming. Parents should not hesitate to voice their concerns to the medical team and seek additional help for themselves, if necessary. Although no parents want to find out that their child has a chronic disease, making the diagnosis has positive aspects. Diagnosis is the first step in starting treatment, and it allows for the education of the child and the family about this illness.

To help you and your family understand and accept the diagnosis of IBD, your child's doctor needs to be aware of how your family works. Doctors need to know, for example, who the primary caregiver of the sick child will be (or whether there will be more than one primary caregiver).

The primary caregiver will be the person who fills prescriptions, gives the child medications, and makes sure the child gets to all follow-up appointments.

The sick child's siblings need to learn about IBD. It is an unfortunate fact that doctors, and even parents, often ignore siblings when bad things happen. Involving siblings when they are at an appropriate age has several good results. First, it ensures constant communication among all family members, and thus the family works better as a unit. Second, it tends to make the child with IBD less different—the child is not singled out from his siblings. The third advantage is that including siblings avoids them feeling left out. Siblings of a child with IBD often feel isolated.

For most people and most ages, having information and knowing what to expect reduces anxiety, allows the child and family to feel more in control of the disease, and makes it possible for the family to work with health care providers as a team.

When surveyed, teenagers with IBD say it is very important for the doctor to take time when giving them information about the diagnosis of IBD. These teenagers feel that the doctor should not appear rushed when giving them the information. They are also virtually unanimous in saying that they prefer having the doctor talk directly to them about IBD, rather than talking to them through their parents. In that direct communication process, they want the doctor to provide easy-to-understand information about the disease and what to expect.

Some parents prefer to hear the news of this diagnosis first so that they can help their children understand. The doctor will want to establish a good relationship with every member of the family and discuss the diagnosis and management of IBD in a way that works well for all of them.

Regardless of where you hear the diagnosis (in the doctor's office or in the recovery room, for example), take the time to let the information sink in, and be sure your doctor answers any questions you have. The discussion should take place privately, not in a hallway outside the child's hospital room. You should also let your doctor know if you are too tired or stressed to receive the news. If you (or your child) do not feel you can handle any news at the moment, ask the doctor to talk to you a little later.

Doctors should discuss certain specific issues with parent and child when giving the diagnosis of IBD. They may not address all these concerns at the first visit, but they should cover them all within the first few visits after the diagnosis:

- Your child's doctor should give your family information about important features of the disease, particularly definitions of inflammatory bowel disease, Crohn's disease, and ulcerative colitis.
- The doctor should tell you who the members of the health care team are, what their roles are, and how to reach them.
- Your child's health care team, including the doctor, should address your family's concerns and fears and answer your questions in a way that helps you and your child feel you have good control over the disease.

Most families have several key concerns when they learn the diagnosis of IBD (see chapters 15–19). Usually these concerns involve the following:

- fear of hospitals, medications, and surgery
- the effect of IBD on school participation or participation in sports or other activities
- fear of accidents at school or in other public places, and concern about inability to play with friends outside the home
- a child's feeling that the disease was his fault, and that he is a burden on others
- feeling isolated or "different"

If your child's health care team does not address these concerns, be sure to ask about them.

7

Laboratory Testing

Routine and specialized laboratory tests are regularly used to help make the diagnosis of and manage IBD. Some tests are helpful in telling the difference between IBD and other conditions that have similar symptoms. Others can be used to tell the difference between Crohn's disease and ulcerative colitis. Tests can also help doctors evaluate how active the disease is, or watch for disease-related complications and side effects of treatments. Test results are generally not used by themselves but are taken together with the overall condition and symptoms of the individual patient.

IBD activity is usually monitored based on overall signs and symptoms, such as whether the child is having abdominal pain, diarrhea, blood in the stool, weight loss, or poor weight gain. The activity of the disease is also monitored by assessing the child's well-being in areas such as energy and activity levels, school attendance, and participation in sports and social functions.

Laboratory tests are helpful in disease management, too, because inflammation produces changes that can be measured in the blood and in the stool. Laboratory test results usually return to normal when the IBD is not active. Once disease-related blood and stool test results are known for a particular child (called baseline results), changes in those specific results can generally be used to monitor the activity of the child's IBD. Test results offer a way of assessing whether your child's IBD is active or inactive in addition to how she is acting and feeling.

Laboratory test results, which are not dependent on the child's understanding or opinion of the disease, can be particularly helpful in making treatment decisions about children and teenagers who are reluctant to discuss their symptoms. They are also helpful in children who feel well and have few, if any, symptoms but who still have considerable continuing intestinal inflammation.

Routine lab tests are usually ordered because they

- can help distinguish between IBD and noninflammatory conditions that have similar symptoms;
- provide a sense of how severe the inflammation is; and
- allow the doctor to identify which of the blood tests will be useful to follow in monitoring disease activity in a particular child.

Routine Blood Analysis

The results of routine blood tests generally show the following changes from the normal baseline when inflammation is active:

- white blood cell count (WBC) increases
- platelet count (Plt) increases
- erythrocyte sedimentation rate (ESR) increases
- C-reactive protein (CRP) increases
- red blood cell count (RBC) decreases (commonly referred to as anemia); the two most common measures of red blood cell numbers are the hemoglobin (Hgb) and hematocrit (Hct)
- albumin (one of the main blood proteins) decreases

Not all patients have all these abnormalities, and some patients may have normal or near-normal blood test values even though they still have very active IBD. It is also important to recognize that these blood tests are not specific for IBD. They may be abnormal in the face of *any* condition that causes inflammation, including infection.

Stool Studies

Stool culture, microscopic examination, and special testing of the stool all check for potential digestive tract infections. The presence of tiny amounts of blood in the stool is a *nonspecific marker*, which may suggest the presence of inflammation but not what specifically causes it. Similarly, identification of elevated levels of the blood protein *alpha-1-antitrypsin* in the stool may be a sign of injury to the intestinal lining (this protein is resistant to the normal process of protein digestion in the gut). The presence of intact white blood cells in the stool also means inflammation, either from IBD or from infection in the gut. The presence of *lactoferrin* or *calprotectin* (types of proteins) in the stool is a marker of intestinal inflammation. Unfortunately, as with routine blood tests, these stool tests are non-specific and do not necessarily distinguish between intestinal inflammation caused by a bacterial infection and inflammation due to IBD.

Lab Tests to Monitor for Side Effects and Complications

Many of the blood tests used to track disease activity also provide information about potential medication-related side effects. These tests include blood counts and blood tests of how well the liver works (ALT, AST, GGT, bilirubin, alkaline phosphatase). Other important blood tests that check for treatment-related side effects are kidney function tests (BUN and creatinine) and tests of the pancreas (amylase and lipase). Nutritional deficiencies associated with IBD that can be detected through laboratory tests are vitamin levels, such as vitamin D or B12, and levels of minerals, such as zinc and iron.

The usefulness and potential harm of some IBD medications can be related to levels of the drug or to its breakdown products in the person's blood. For biologic medications (drugs made from proteins rather than chemicals), such as infliximab and adalimumab, there are also tests to check for antibodies to the drug (proteins that a person's body might make that counteract the medication). Drug antibodies may lead to the medicine not working as well, or to the development of an allergic reaction in the person receiving the medicine. Checking blood levels or drug antibodies is important for the following medicines:

- cyclosporine
- tacrolimus
- 6-mercaptopurine (6-MP)

- azathioprine
- biologic medications (e.g., infliximab, adalimumab)

Measuring drug levels or the levels of breakdown products can help doctors evaluate whether specific symptoms are due to side effects of the drug or to ongoing disease activity. Measuring drug levels can also help assess whether the child is taking the correct dose of the medication. It can identify whether a child may be having problems with drug absorption or with compliance (taking the medicine as directed). Constant disease activity despite the right drug levels in the blood may be a sign that the particular treatment is not effective for the child. The family and the doctor may want to explore different treatments rather than wait weeks or months to see what happens. It is possible to test a child ahead of time to find out whether he is able to break down 6-MP and azathioprine; if he is not, then different medications will be more effective for that child.

IBD-Specific Laboratory Tests

In the last section, we mentioned antibodies to drugs that can make them less effective or lead to an allergic reaction. Antibodies are also an important component in IBD. They are proteins that the immune system produces to fight infections and unfamiliar material that enters the body. When antibodies fight infections, they cause inflammation. The search for the trigger of abnormal inflammation that is typical in IBD has led to the discovery of several specific antibodies. These antibodies are present in the blood of many people with CD or UC but are usually not present in children without IBD, which makes them markers for the disease. The most commonly identified markers are pANCA and ASCA. Newer antibody tests have also been developed such as anti–outer membrane protein C (OmpC) and anti-CBir1.

As we have discussed and as you may know firsthand, diagnosing pediatric IBD is challenging. This is why the search for accurate, noninvasive markers of IBD has been stepped up. These antibody markers, when they are found in diagnostic test results, may help doctors recognize IBD more quickly. They may also indicate whether a child has CD, UC, or some other condition. Yet, these laboratory tests are *not* specific for IBD. At times, the detected levels may be falsely elevated in children without IBD (*false positive*), or the results may be negative when a child actually has IBD. Therefore, these blood tests are *not* a substitute for other blood and imaging studies and colonoscopy.

The IBD marker tests involve only blood tests, and they do not require putting a scope or other instrument inside the body. Talk with your child's doctor about whether antibody tests can be helpful in your child's particular case. Future research will focus on identifying more of these antibodies to improve our ability to diagnose IBD with confidence.

8

Imaging Studies

This chapter describes some of the imaging studies used most often to diagnose IBD and to monitor its potential complications. Imaging studies use x-rays, sound waves, or other methods to take pictures of the inside of the body.

Abdominal Plain Film

The abdominal plain film is a simple x-ray picture of the abdomen (belly area), taken when your child is either lying flat on the x-ray table or standing up. This picture can show how much air and stool is in the intestine. The pattern of air and stool can be helpful in showing whether your child is constipated. The doctor can also learn from this x-ray whether there might be a blockage or a hole in the intestine.

This type of x-ray is sometimes called the KUB, which stands for kidneys, ureters, and bladder. The x-ray is supposed to include the kidneys, ureters (the tubes that go from the kidneys to the bladder), and the bladder, but in reality, these three organs usually do not show well on the abdominal plain film.

Upper Gastrointestinal and Small Bowel Series

The upper GI and small bowel series are x-ray pictures of the abdomen performed after the patient drinks liquid barium. *Barium* is a type of chemical that tastes a little like chalk, but sometimes the taste can be improved by adding chocolate or strawberry flavoring to the liquid. Still, many children find drinking the barium difficult, and they may require some coaxing. On x-ray, the barium shows up white, while the rest of the body is mostly gray or black.

The contrast of white as it goes through the digestive tract gives a picture of the size, shape, and location of

- the esophagus (the tube leading from the throat to the stomach),
- the stomach, and
- the small intestine.

This test shows pictures of what the inside of the digestive tract looks like, but it does not show the actual lining and muscles of the tract. The results are generally normal in ulcerative colitis, but the images can show changes in the small intestine that would suggest Crohn's disease. The test is useful in detecting a shaggy lining or separation of parts of the intestine. Shaggy linings and separations can indicate swelling and irritation.

The upper GI and small bowel series can also show other problems:

- ulceration
- narrowing (stricture) in the small intestine
- an enlarged intestinal segment that could mean there is a blockage
- a fistula (an abnormal connection between loops of the intestine)

This study typically requires fasting (nothing by mouth) for about 4 hours before the test. Since the goal of the test is to examine the entire small intestine, the procedure may take 3 hours or longer (with periods of x-raying alternating with periods of waiting). At some point, the radiologist may push on the child's abdomen to help separate the loops of intestine to achieve better x-ray pictures.

Barium Enema

The barium enema is an x-ray of the colon (the large intestine). The barium is squirted up into the rectum (which connects the colon to the anus) through a tube inserted into the anal opening. Under pressure, the barium goes through the entire colon, all the way to its beginning (called the cecum). The white barium gives a picture of the size, shape, and appearance of the colon. It outlines what the inside of the colon looks like but does not make a picture of the actual lining and muscles of the colon. This test is useful in detecting a shaggy lining (which would indicate swelling and irritation).

The barium enema can also show other problems:

- ulceration
- narrowing (stricture) in the intestine
- an enlarged intestinal segment that could mean there is a blockage
- a fistula (an abnormal connection between loops of the intestine)

Sometimes the barium goes into the terminal ileum, the part of the small intestine that connects to the colon. When this happens, the doctors can see that area as well. Although the barium enema used to be a common test in patients with suspected IBD, it is rarely needed now that colonoscopies (see chapter 9) are widely performed in children.

Computed Tomography

Computed tomography, or CT scan—sometimes referred to as a CAT scan—is a special kind of x-ray that converts computer images of the body into pictures. In this test, the patient drinks a large amount of a special liquid dye (called an *oral contrast*) that helps show the size, shape, and location of the GI tract. Usually, the radiologist also injects a different contrast material into the veins (*intravenous [IV] contrast*). IV contrast shows more clearly the features of the solid organs (like the liver and kidneys). The patient lies inside a short cylinder that houses a camera, which takes pictures from different angles. The camera usually makes noise as it moves inside the cylinder.

A CT scan of the abdomen and pelvis, with oral and IV contrast dyes, can provide a great deal of information about the GI tract, including

- the presence of an abscess (a pocket of infection)
- the possibility of appendicitis
- whether the bowel wall is too thick (indicating the presence of swelling and irritation of the intestine)
- a narrow or enlarged segment of bowel
- a fistula

The CT scan shows pictures of the lining and muscles of the GI tract as well as some pictures of the inside of the tract. Other solid organs, including the liver, spleen, gallbladder, pancreas, and kidneys, are also visible on the CT scan. The test further shows normal and abnormal lymph nodes, as well as tumors in the abdomen.

Ultrasound

The ultrasound uses sound waves to make images, much like a submarine uses sonar to make a picture of the bottom of the ocean. The sound waves are aimed at, and bounce off, the intestines and other organs in the abdomen. These organs include the gallbladder, pancreas, kidneys, and appendix. The patient does not have to drink any contrast dye or have anything put in the rectum. No intravenous (IV) liquids are necessary. A technician will spread a gel over the abdomen, and the ultrasound device painlessly touches the skin, sliding over the gel.

The ultrasound shows the appearance of the muscles of the digestive tract but not the inside of the tract. This test is useful in detecting gallstones, pancreatitis, kidney stones, or kidney blockage. Ultrasound can also point to the possibility of appendicitis, and show whether the bowel wall is thick and swollen, possibly as a result of inflammation.

Magnetic Resonance Imaging

A magnetic resonance imaging (MRI) test uses magnets to excite molecules (tiny particles) in the cells of the body. Similar to what happens in preparing for a CT scan, the patient has to drink a large amount of oral contrast liquid dye, which helps show the size, shape, and location of the GI tract; a different contrast given into the vein is also used. MRI of the abdomen (also called *magnetic resonance enterography*, or MRE) can evaluate the intestines as well as other organs, such as the liver and pancreas. Since MRI does not expose the patient to any harmful radiation, it is becoming an increasingly popular imaging study to evaluate children with IBD.

Some patients feel uncomfortable while inside the tube, because they do not like being enclosed in a tight space. Many young children receive sedation (medicine to make them sleepy) before an MRI test. Sedation makes children feel more comfortable, and allows them to hold still for the test.

Bone Age X-Ray

The bone age x-ray evaluates how mature the child's bones are and how much more growing she is able to do. The bones of the hands and wrists in children have growth centers that develop and then disappear into the bones. Bones look different as the child ages as well as when the bones are fully grown. The bone age x-ray compares the age of the bones with the age of your child. When the bone age is less than your child's age, there is more time for the bones to keep growing. A short child who has a bone age less than the child's age is likely to keep growing and has the potential to catch up and grow to the height that she was meant to be based on her genes.

Bone Density Scan

A bone density scan, also called dual-energy x-ray absorptiometry (DXA or DEXA), is a special form of x-ray technology that measures bone mineral density and that is used to diagnose low bone density (osteopenia or osteoporosis). Decreased bone density is common in adults with IBD and can be seen in children and adolescents with IBD as well. Considerably decreased bone density can increase the risk of broken bones (fractures).

Poor nutrition, low vitamin and mineral levels, little exercise or few weight-bearing activities, or use of corticosteroids (such as prednisone) can increase the risk of low bone density. The bone density scan uses a very small dose of radiation and is most often performed on the lower spine and hips. The patient lies on a table that has an "arm" suspended overhead. The test is painless and takes 10 or 15 minutes.

Tests for Special Purposes

Newly developed imaging tests can help in the diagnosis of inflammatory bowel disease and its related complications. This section highlights three such techniques, which make it possible to see areas that were previously reachable only through invasive endoscopic procedures (see chapter 9), or through surgical exploration. These special imaging procedures are becoming more common as doctors seek noninvasive ways of evaluating patients. None of these methods, however, gives doctors the opportunity to take biopsies (tissue samples for examination) or to treat strictures (narrowed areas in the intestines).

Capsule Endoscopy

Beyond the first part of the small intestine (duodenum) and near the last part (terminal ileum), the rest of the small intestine (8 to 16 feet) is usually impossible to reach with a standard endoscope. Wireless capsule endoscopy is a technique of viewing the entire small intestine with a video camera housed in a small pill (a pill camera), which is about 1 inch long and half an inch wide. The patient can swallow the capsule, or the doctor can place it in the small intestine using an endoscope. The video capsule is equipped with a camera and a battery that can last many hours.

The capsule transmits continuous video images as it travels through the small intestine. A receiver captures and stores these images. The information is then downloaded into a computer equipped with specialized software, which enables doctors to see the lining of the entire small intestine. They can identify inflamed areas, ulcers, bleeding lesions, and pseudopolyps (inflamed tissue that looks like polyps). Because the patient is wearing multiple circular patches (receivers) over the entire abdomen, the position of these abnormal areas can be pinpointed, and pictures or even video clips can be stored for later examination. The capsule is expelled in a bowel movement and flushed down the toilet.

Magnetic Resonance Cholangiopancreatography

Some patients with IBD develop inflammation and strictures in their bile ducts, inside and outside the liver. This condition is called *primary sclerosing cholangitis* (PSC). PSC normally occurs after IBD is diagnosed, though it sometimes exists before it is known that the child has IBD. Up until a decade ago, the only way to diagnose PSC was through an endoscopy in which a catheter was inserted into the bile ducts. This invasive procedure is called *endoscopic retrograde cholangiopancreatography* (ERCP).

Over the last ten years, examination of the bile ducts inside and outside the liver has been perfected using a special noninvasive imaging technique called *magnetic resonance cholangiopancreatography* (MRCP). MRCP takes advantage of the fact that structures filled with nonmoving or slow-moving fluids, such as bile ducts, appear bright white against a black background in an MRI. This circumstance often makes it unnecessary to perform the more invasive ERCP study. As with regular MRI tests, some children will need sedation for the MRCP.

Virtual Colonoscopy

Improvements in CT techniques, and the use of computer modeling, have allowed radiologists to reconstruct a 3-D model of the colon, called a *CT colonography* (or, more popularly, *virtual colonoscopy*). In adults, the procedure takes about 10 minutes and requires no sedation. Patients lie on their backs while a continuously rotating x-ray beam provides images of the entire colon. The procedure is repeated with the patient on his stomach. A computer program puts these images together in a movielike series of 3-D pictures.

This technique is most useful in detecting colon polyps and screening for colon cancer. At this point, few studies apply CT colonography to the diagnosis of IBD. Strictures and wall thickening, which indicate diffuse inflammation, may be detected using this technique, but flat lesions and the shallow ulcerations that characterize IBD may not be. With continued improvements in resolution and speed, both CT-based and MRI-based computer modeling will likely find greater uses in diagnosing and monitoring children with IBD.

▣ 9

Endoscopic Exams

Endoscopy of the digestive tract is a tool that most people with inflammatory bowel disease are or will become familiar with. It is one of the most commonly used tools to diagnose IBD. Endoscopy involves the use of a specially designed flexible tube containing a camera, called an endoscope, to look inside the intestines. Doctors use endoscopy to diagnose IBD and to help them determine and monitor the treatment of the disease. The special camera enables doctors to see areas of the digestive tract that may be inflamed in patients with IBD or similar conditions. It also helps doctors detect other types of inflammation, such as those caused by excessive stomach acid (reflux), bacterial or viral infections, or medications. This chapter describes endoscopic procedures, including how to prepare for them and what's involved in the recovery period.

Types of Endoscopic Procedures

Four main types of endoscopy are performed in pediatric patients with IBD (figure 9.1).

1. Upper endoscopy, or EGD (esophagogastroduodenoscopy), examines the esophagus, stomach, and upper portion of the small intestine.
2. Colonoscopy looks at the entire colon (large intestine) and often the last part of the small intestine (terminal ileum).

3. Sigmoidoscopy is a limited form of colonoscopy. It examines only the last two parts of the colon: the rectum (very end of the colon) and the sigmoid colon (portion of the colon just above the rectum). Sigmoidoscopy typically requires less sedation time and less preparation than a full colonoscopy.

4. ERCP (endoscopic retrograde cholangiopancreatography) is performed with a specially designed endoscope (called a side-viewing scope) that can evaluate the bile ducts (ducts that drain bile from the liver) and the pancreatic duct (which drains the pancreas).

Each type of endoscopy is performed with an endoscope designed specifically for that procedure. Endoscopes have a channel running through them that doctors can use to wash the bowel or blow in air to improve their view during the test. This channel also enables doctors to pass instruments in and out during the procedure. A pediatric gastroenterologist might pass any of these instruments through the channel:

- biopsy forceps, to obtain a sample of tissue for examination under the microscope
- balloons that can dilate (widen) narrowed areas of the bowel
- needles to inject medicine directly into the bowel wall, including medicine to help control bleeding
- various probes used to stop bleeding or remove abnormal tissue
- snares to remove polyps that may be detected during endoscopy
- brushes that can sample fluid or mucus on the lining to look for infections
- various other specialized forceps, to retrieve both foreign objects and polyps

The Purpose of Endoscopy

Children and adolescents with IBD usually need an endoscopy for one or more of these six reasons:

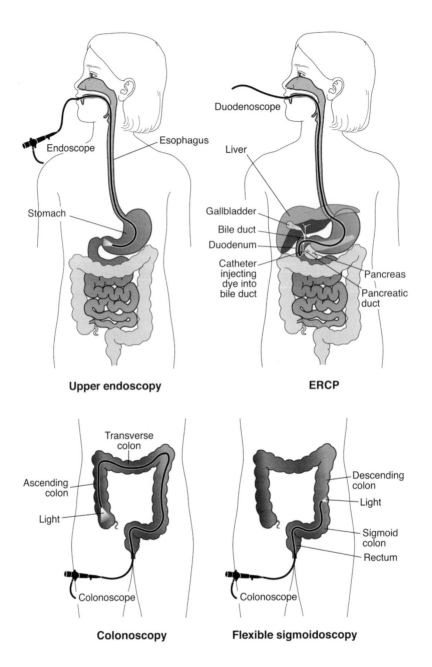

Upper endoscopy

Endoscope
Esophagus
Stomach

ERCP

Duodenoscope
Liver
Gallbladder
Bile duct
Duodenum
Catheter injecting dye into bile duct
Pancreas
Pancreatic duct

Colonoscopy

Transverse colon
Ascending colon
Light
Colonoscope

Flexible sigmoidoscopy

Descending colon
Light
Sigmoid colon
Rectum
Colonoscope

1. to confirm a diagnosis of IBD
2. to evaluate (or reevaluate) how much of the bowel is inflamed, and how severely it is affected
3. to help the physician determine whether a change in treatment is needed
4. to treat symptoms or complications of IBD, such as bleeding
5. to treat a specific problem—for example, to widen a stricture (narrow area)
6. to look for precancerous changes

Biopsies are taken from all segments of the gastrointestinal (GI) tract and are very important in deciding whether the condition is ulcerative colitis, Crohn's disease, or inflammation due to another reason. Biopsies are also important in assessing the severity of the inflammation. In long-standing disease (ten years' duration or more), biopsies done during a colonoscopy can detect the early changes of colon cancer.

Having endoscopy may be uncomfortable or even painful because the endoscope is pushed around the turns in the intestine. After the procedure, bloating that results from filling the colon with air (so that the doctor can see the lining) adds to the discomfort. Doctors and parents understand how important it is to make this procedure as pain-free as possible for children with IBD, because they will very likely need other endoscopies as the years go by. Younger children as well as anxious teenagers and young adults are given general anesthesia by an anesthesiologist. For older, cooperative, and

---

Figure 9.1. Endoscopic procedures in inflammatory bowel disease. In upper endoscopy, a long flexible tube is passed into the mouth and is used to examine the esophagus, stomach, and upper small intestine (*top left*). A modified version of this procedure, called endoscopic retrograde cholangiopancreatography (ERCP), can be used to evaluate the bile ducts and pancreas (*top right*). Lower GI endoscopy is done by inserting a tube through the anus and examining the entire colon (colonoscopy; *bottom left*) or a portion of the colon (flexible sigmoidoscopy; *bottom right*).

less anxious children, a technique called *conscious sedation* may be used. In conscious sedation, the child is given medication to make him sleepy and comfortable during the procedure, but an anesthesiologist is typically not present. The medication for conscious sedation is usually administered by the gastroenterologist and nurses performing the procedure.

For an upper endoscopy, no preparation of the intestine is needed. But most people who have had a colonoscopy agree that the most difficult part of the process is preparing the colon before the procedure. The purpose of the colon preparation is to remove fecal material (stool) from the colon so that the lining of the large intestine can be examined effectively. Preparation can be done in different ways (see below), but there is no easy way to clean out the colon. Cleaning that cannot be done successfully at home may have to be done in the hospital. Procedures may be canceled and rescheduled if the clean-out is not adequate.

Parents need to understand the options for preparing the bowel and sedating their child. Discussing these options with the doctor will minimize stress and ensure that the special needs of the child are met.

Although endoscopy is generally a very safe procedure, known risks include inadvertently putting a hole in the intestine (perforation) or causing additional bleeding or an infection. In addition, the sedation or anesthesia itself carries a small risk of side effects. The endoscopist is responsible for explaining these risks to the family and obtaining their written consent for the procedure. The consent form indicates that the risks of the procedure have been discussed with the parent.

How Is Endoscopy Done in Children and Adolescents with IBD?

Doctors with special training in pediatric gastroenterology, including pediatric endoscopy, perform the procedure. As noted above, to minimize discomfort, patients are usually under some form of sedation or anesthesia (deeply relaxed or sleeping).

In EGD and ERCP, the endoscope passes through the mouth into the esophagus (the pipe that takes food from the throat into the stomach), and from the esophagus into the stomach and then the small intestine. Standard upper endoscopes can pass only into the first portion of the small intestine, known as the duodenum. An additional 19 to 26 feet (6 to 8 meters) of small intestine are not reachable by standard upper endoscopy. The doctor may use a longer endoscope, an *enteroscope*, to examine the second part of the small intestine, known as the *jejunum*, especially for patients who are thought to have small bowel disease farther down in the intestine. In ERCP, which usually involves injecting a special dye into the bile or pancreatic ducts, the endoscope passes into the second portion of the duodenum, where the bile and pancreatic ducts drain into the bowel.

In colonoscopy and sigmoidoscopy, the endoscope enters through the anus into the rectum and from there passes throughout the remainder of the colon. The colon is a long and winding organ shaped something like a question mark, measuring 3 to 6 feet (1 to 2 meters) in an adult. Colonoscopy is more difficult to perform than an EGD and often takes longer.

During a colonoscopy in a patient with known or suspected IBD, most pediatric gastroenterologists attempt to enter the very end of the small intestine, known as the terminal ileum. Because the terminal ileum is the portion of the bowel that is commonly involved with CD, examining this area is important when trying to distinguish between UC and CD.

Preparation and Procedure

Most endoscopic examinations are elective rather than emergency procedures, which means that the doctor, patient, and family are able to schedule the procedure. If elective, the procedure is performed when the patient does not have any active breathing problems or infections and is in stable condition. Patients (or their parents) should tell their doctors if illness symptoms develop before the procedure, such as a cough, runny nose, fever, or other problems. The doctor may want to reschedule the procedure for another day, to reduce the risk of complications, such as infection.

In some patients who are ill (either in the hospital or at home), the procedure may need to be performed despite the illness symptoms. For example, these exams may be needed to diagnose IBD, or to assist in the treatment of a patient who is becoming increasingly ill because of her IBD. The procedures may be necessary to treat children with complications of IBD. Patients and their families should understand the possible increased risk connected with having these procedures done while the child is ill. Discuss with the doctor any concerns you have.

EGD, ERCP, and Capsule Endoscopy

For most patients with IBD, the only required preparation for EGD, ERCP, and capsule endoscopy is fasting (no food or drink). The length of fasting is determined by the patient's age. You should check with your child's doctor for the appropriate fasting time for your child. If your child takes daily medications, such as medicines for diabetes, seizures, or other chronic conditions, you should check with his doctor for specific instructions. Some medications should not be taken on the day of the procedure, and the dosage of some medicines may need to change on the day of the test. If your child has a heart condition or a prosthetic device, check with his doctor for specific instructions regarding preventive antibiotics before or after the procedure. Some patients who are having an ERCP will receive antibiotics before the procedure because they are at an increased risk of infection due to their underlying condition. Blood tests or x-rays may also be required before the procedure, if the doctor thinks they would be helpful.

Colonoscopy and Sigmoidoscopy

A colonoscopy requires fasting as well as bowel clean-out before the procedure. The bowel is cleaned out for three reasons.

1. Bowel cleaning in advance allows the doctor to effectively examine the lining of the large intestine for abnormalities.
2. A clean bowel makes the procedure easier to perform.
3. A clean bowel reduces the risk of complications for the patient.

Doctors may choose to cancel the colonoscopy in a patient who has not had a good bowel cleaning. Although doctors have some ability to wash the bowel during the colonoscopy, this washing does not make up for an unprepared bowel.

Bowel-cleaning routines differ among medical centers and even among doctors at the same center. There are different routines because no one "best" method works in all patients, is easy to take, and is completely effective. Bowel preparation usually includes taking in only clear liquids (water, clear broth, etc.) for one to two days before the procedure, as well as adding laxatives. Laxatives are medicines (prescription or over the counter) that can encourage bowel movements or make them softer. They are given on the day of, or one to two days before, the procedure. Common medicines used for this purpose include polyethylene glycol and drugs that contain magnesium (such as magnesium citrate), bisacodyl, senna, or sodium phosphate. These laxatives are usually in liquid form, although some are available as pills. In addition, some doctors tell their patients to have enemas, either on the evening before or on the morning of the procedure. The specific bowel-cleaning procedure is based on the patient's age and weight. A different procedure can be used if the first one does not work as expected. Even in patients who have diarrhea, a specific bowel-cleaning procedure is usually required.

Flexible sigmoidoscopy generally requires a modification of the colonoscopy routine outlined above. In some patients who are having significant diarrhea, additional bowel-cleansing medications are not required for a flexible sigmoidoscopy. If patients will be sedated for the procedure, fasting beforehand is necessary.

Sedation and Anesthesia

There are many types of sedation that a child can receive for the endoscopic procedure. Medicines for sedation reduce discomfort during the exam and make the child forget the experience when it is over. Doctors generally group the level of sedation a patient will get into one of three categories: conscious sedation, deep sedation, or general anesthesia.

Patients receiving conscious sedation can respond to commands during the endoscopy but generally do not remember the procedure or experience pain during it. Patients who are under deep sedation or general anesthesia cannot respond to commands, do not remember the procedure, and do not experience pain during it. Depending on the medicine used, however, patients under deep sedation or general anesthesia may take longer to wake up after the endoscopy than those under conscious sedation. With deep sedation or general anesthesia, usually an anesthesiologist is involved in the procedure, which may increase the cost and time it takes.

What to Expect during the Procedure

Depending on the endoscopy method, patients may lie on their back, on their left side, or, for ERCP, on their stomach. Those undergoing an EGD under conscious sedation may experience some very brief gagging during the procedure. Most patients do not remember this. Those undergoing colonoscopy may experience abdominal cramping or distension (feeling full) during the endoscopy. This discomfort is due to the air the doctor blows into the bowel to help the scope pass and to make the intestinal lining easier to see. The doctor can remove some of the air when removing the scope, but the patient frequently needs to pass the air (pass gas) after the procedure is done. This will relieve the feeling of fullness or bloating.

Cramping can also occur during these procedures because the endoscope forms loops. Pediatric gastroenterologists are particularly aware of the discomfort associated with loop formation, and they try to minimize it if possible, but some looping can still occur. Patients may be turned to one side or the other during the procedure to help reduce looping. The cramping due to looping is usually short lived.

Biopsies are not painful. In fact, if a conscious patient were not told that a biopsy was being performed, she would probably not be able to tell when the biopsy was happening. Pain in the bowel is caused by distension, not the small pinching that occurs during biopsies. Although patients and families are often most concerned about what biopsies will feel like, this part of the endoscopic procedure is usually the least uncomfortable.

The feeling of gagging (with upper endoscopy) or cramping (with lower endoscopy) usually improves when the scope is withdrawn in the second half of the endoscopic exam. This is when treatment procedures such as biopsies or polyp removal are typically done.

What to Expect after the Procedure

EGD

Patients may be nauseated after an upper endoscopy and may have a sore throat. Some patients may need intravenous (IV) fluids or an antinausea medication after the procedure. Generally, though, these problems go away with little treatment. Severe chest pain can develop after an upper endoscopy, and patients or family members should notify their doctor immediately if the child develops significant chest pain after endoscopy, or if he has other symptoms as described below (under ERCP).

ERCP

Patients who have had an ERCP are at risk for complications after the procedure, including pancreatitis, infection with or without fever, and gastrointestinal bleeding if a treatment was performed during the endoscopy. Pancreatitis is usually associated with severe abdominal pain. Seek immediate medical attention if your child develops

- significant abdominal pain
- fever
- vomiting of blood
- blood in the stool or black stools
- dizziness or lightheadedness

Colonoscopy and Flexible Sigmoidoscopy

After the procedure, many patients experience some degree of nausea, fullness, or bloating. As with EGD, some patients may need IV fluids or an antinausea medication after the examination. Generally, though, these problems disappear with little treatment. If your child develops significant abdominal pain, increased blood in her bowel movements, or fever, seek immediate medical attention.

Procedures Performed under Sedation or General Anesthesia

In addition to infection, bleeding, and pain from the endoscopy, patients may experience side effects from the anesthesia or sedation, or from the way it was given. (A side effect does not necessarily indicate a problem with the procedure or with the anesthesia, however.) Common side effects include sleepiness, nausea, and vomiting. If your child had a breathing tube in her throat during the endoscopy, she may experience a sore throat for a few days. Patients are generally advised not to return to work or school on the day of an endoscopic procedure with sedation. Those who are old enough to drive should not do so until the day after the endoscopy. Your child should not engage in activities that require a high degree of coordination until the next day, when the effects of anesthesia and sedation will have worn off.

Contact your child's doctor immediately if your child develops any of the following symptoms after endoscopy:

- breathing difficulties
- chest or abdominal pain
- fever
- prolonged vomiting
- increased blood in the stool
- vomiting blood
- any other concerns

The above listing is not all inclusive. Ask your child's doctor for instructions to follow before *and after* any endoscopy. If you are unable to contact the doctor and are concerned about symptoms that occur after the procedure, take your child to the emergency room for evaluation.

Risks and Complications of Endoscopy

As with any medical procedure, there are risks associated with endoscopy. If your child receives medications to sedate him on any level, these medications and the way they are given also carry risks. Discuss the potential risks and complications with the doctors who will be performing the endoscopic exam and with the anesthesiologist, if an anesthesiologist will be involved.

The risks and potential complications of endoscopy include

- a hole in the intestinal tract (perforation)
- increased or new bleeding
- infection
- breathing problems
- a bad reaction to medication

The degree of risk varies depending on several factors:

- the child's symptoms
- how much of the bowel is affected by the disease
- the child's general health
- the type of procedure
- how well the bowel is cleaned out (for colonoscopy and flexible sigmoidoscopy)
- whether a more difficult procedure is being performed during the endoscopy (for example, dilating or stretching a portion of the bowel that is narrowed)

In general, the risk of a healthy and well-prepared patient experiencing some type of complication in a normal upper endoscopy or colonoscopy is between 1 in 1,000 cases to 1 in 10,000 cases. Endoscopic risk also depends on the experience of the doctor performing the test. Patients and their families should ask their doctors about their experience with pediatric endoscopy. Ideally the doctor has a great deal of experience and a very low complication rate.

You can help decrease the risk of complications by telling doctors about any other medical problems your child has. Your child's doctor also needs to know about any problems your child has had with procedures or sedation as well as any related family medical history. You should also alert the doctor if your child develops illness symptoms such as cough, fever, or congestion prior to his scheduled procedure.

Your child must strictly follow the doctor's orders for preparations before the procedure, such as having nothing by mouth (fasting) for a period prior to the endoscopy. Patients who eat beforehand instead of fasting as directed risk vomiting during the endoscopic exam. The vomitus may enter the airway and cause severe pneumonia. Maintaining strict pre-procedure fasting is especially important with young children who, not understanding the potentially severe consequences, may try to sneak food. Similarly, a patient's failure to take the fully prescribed bowel preparation prolongs the procedure and increases the difficulty of the endoscopy, the likelihood of missing an important finding, and the risk of complications, such as a perforation.

Pediatric gastrointestinal endoscopy is a developing field in which significant advances have been made. These advances will continue in the years to come. At this time, endoscopy and endoscopic biopsy are the standard tools for diagnosing CD or UC.

Patients with IBD will likely need more than one endoscopic procedure in their lifetime. Doctors and nurses are working with patients and their families to make these important procedures as safe and easy to tolerate as possible while retaining their usefulness. Endoscopic treatment procedures are also performed on children with IBD. In many cases, the availability of pediatric therapeutic endoscopy (treatments through endoscopy) has reduced the need for surgery in children with UC or CD.

Part III
Treating IBD

▣ 10

Medical Treatments

Currently, no medical therapies can "cure" Crohn's disease or ulcerative colitis, but many medications can keep inflammation at bay, allowing children to feel as well as they did before they were diagnosed with IBD. The goals of treatment are to quickly bring the disease under control (induce remission) and to keep it controlled in the long term (maintain remission). A trusting relationship between the child, the family, and the health care team is extremely important for achieving the goals of treatment. Equally important is close follow-up and monitoring with the IBD-treating doctor, encouraging open communication in both directions.

Inducing and Maintaining Remission

Periods of increased disease activity (flares) are characteristic of IBD and are considered part of its "natural history." The goal for IBD disease management is finding effective *induction* treatment, and subsequently putting the disease into *remission*. When disease is in remission, the symptoms of the disease, such as diarrhea, pain, bleeding, poor appetite, and tiredness, disappear. Just as important, healing the lining of the intestine allows for optimal health in the long term. With disease remission, nutritional status also improves, supporting normal growth as well as unimpeded development in puberty. The health care team can check whether the disease is active or in remission through physical exams, which include tracking growth and development; laboratory testing, including blood and stool tests; and repeating endoscopy when needed.

The most important goal of treatment is to provide as complete a remission as possible, to the point where the child feels well and functions to her optimal potential. Another increasingly important goal of treatment is to achieve *mucosal healing*, which means that endoscopic evaluation of the GI tract shows that it is visibly normal in appearance and ideally that even the biopsies of the intestine also look normal under the microscope. Mucosal healing has been associated with sustained clinical remission, improved growth, decreased hospitalization, and decreased risk of surgery. Thus, achieving complete remission and mucosal healing are vital concepts. Too many children and their families settle for feeling "okay, I guess." Feeling this way, short of what may be truly possible, is not the definition of remission!

After inducing remission, the next goal of treatment is to form a plan that will keep the disease in remission. This is the *maintenance* treatment. The ideal medication to maintain remission will keep the lining of the intestine healed and therefore ward off flares of disease, possible hospitalizations, and surgeries, with few, if any, side effects. The optimal maintenance medication should work well enough to keep the child from requiring any further treatment with steroids.

Medications Used for Treating IBD

Most of the medications prescribed for IBD may be used for both induction therapy and maintenance therapy (table 10.1). Your child's physician will decide which medications to prescribe initially depending on the severity of your child's symptoms. Medications can be administered orally (by mouth); intravenously (through a needle in the vein); intramuscularly (by injection—a shot—in the muscle); subcutaneously (by injection under the skin); or rectally (by enema or suppository).

- Oral medications in general can exert their effects *systemically* (throughout the body) if they are absorbed through the lining of the intestines into the bloodstream.

Table 10.1
Treatments for inducing and maintaining remission

	Induction	Maintenance
5-Aminosalicylates (5-ASA)	+	+
Corticosteroids	+	−
Immunomodulators	−	+
Antibiotics	+	+
Biologics	+	+
Nutrition	+	+

- Some oral medications are designed to become active only when in contact with certain parts of the intestine. They are able to stay largely within the bowel and are poorly absorbed into the bloodstream because of their chemical structures or coatings. These special features enable the drug to target its effects to specific regions of the intestinal tract.
- Rectal preparations tend to be similar to those given by mouth, but they are used to treat inflammation in the last part of the colon (closest to the anus) such as the sigmoid colon and rectum. Rather than having to travel through about 25 feet of intestine to reach and become active at their destination, these medications are delivered straight to the site needing their action.
- Medications injected into muscle, skin, or veins work throughout the body (systemically).

In this chapter, we describe IBD medications and treatments in the order in which they appear in table 10.1.

5-Aminosalicylates

The 5-aminosalicylate (5-ASA) drugs include some of the oldest medications used to treat IBD. The generic names for these drugs are sulfasalazine, mesalamine, olsalazine, and balsalazide. These medications are anti-inflammatory medications chemically related to aspirin that act on the lining of the intestine. There are rectal as well as oral formulations of 5-ASA drugs. In addition, some preparations release the active drug at different levels of the small and large intestines. These options make it possible for your child's doctor to select the best preparation depending on which area of the bowel the disease is affecting. Studies, as well as clinical experience, show that these medications can be used for induction in patients who have mild disease. In addition, 5-ASAs are safe and effective maintenance medications in ulcerative colitis, as well as in select patients with mild Crohn's disease.

The 5-ASAs are the mainstay of maintenance treatment in mild to moderate UC. When given by mouth, they can provide long-term remission. Suppositories deliver medication straight to the rectum, and enemas deliver the medicine to the lower part of the large intestine (left colon). These forms can be used long term or periodically for breakthrough symptoms.

5-ASAs can also be used at times for long-term maintenance in mild CD. Oral preparations deliver the active medication to the small and large intestines. Therefore, these medications can be used for multiple disease locations. The different applications of various 5-ASA drugs are summarized in table 10.2 and described below.

Sulfasalazine

Sulfasalazine was the first 5-ASA drug used successfully to treat UC and CD of the colon. It has been in use for IBD since the 1940s. Sulfasalazine is taken by mouth and is available in both coated and uncoated tablet forms. A pharmacist can make a liquid preparation for children who are unable to swallow tablets. About 25 percent of the drug is absorbed from the small intestine into the bloodstream. The remainder passes into the colon, where normal bacteria break down the medication into its two components, 5-ASA and sulfapyridine. The sulfapyridine molecule acts only as a carrier to deliver the active portion, 5-ASA, to the colon. Most of

Table 10.2
Pill and rectal forms of the 5-aminosalicylates

Pill (sustained or pH- [acid-] sensitive release)

    Mesalamine: specially coated tablets or granules in capsules

Pill (bacterial enzyme [azoreductase] release)

    Sulfasalazine: mesalamine linked to a sulfa antibiotic (sulfapyridine)

    Balsalazide: mesalamine linked to an inactive carrier molecule

    Olsalazine: two mesalamine molecules linked together

Rectal

    Mesalamine: rectal suspension enema or suppository

Note: Most aminosalicylate medications are taken by mouth, and some of them are also available in enema or suppository form. This table lists some of the different forms of these medications.

the active 5-ASA remains in contact with the inflamed lining of the colon before it passes from the body in stool.

Virtually all the information we have about treating IBD with different types of 5-ASA is derived from adult experience. Sulfasalazine is often effective in mildly to moderately active UC or CD of the colon. It is also the one 5-ASA that helps treat joint inflammation, which sometimes accompanies IBD. Symptoms of mild colitis should disappear in most patients within three to four weeks of starting treatment. Success rates with sulfasalazine are dose related—the higher the dose, the more likely the beneficial response. But higher doses tend to result in various side effects. The sulfa in its chemical structure is responsible for most of the side effects caused by sulfasalazine. The most common of these side effects, occurring in about 15 to 30 percent of patients, include decreased appetite, headaches (especially in the front part of the head), nausea, and vomiting. Rarely, sulfasalazine can worsen bloody diarrhea or cause rash, fever, or signs of severe allergic reaction. Sulfasalazine can reduce the absorption of folic acid (one of the B vitamins) from the small intestine into the bloodstream and can therefore cause anemia. To prevent this complication, children should take supplemental folic acid while on this medication. Sulfasalazine can cause temporary and reversible infertility in males by its effects on sperm. (This problem disappears when the patient stops taking the medication.)

Sulfa-Free 5-ASA Medications

The dose-limiting side effects of sulfasalazine led to the development of sulfa-free 5-ASA medications including mesalamine, balsalazide, and olsalazine. The benefit of these medications is similar to that of sulfasalazine. Greater improvement with mesalamine is noted with higher doses, which are more well tolerated because mesalamine medications do not contain sulfa. It is therefore possible to start treatment, or gradually increase treatment, with higher dosages, based on the patient's need.

5-ASAs also help sustain remission in patients with mild to moderate colitis that results from either CD or UC. The treatment has minimal side effects. In CD, some studies suggest that treatment with mesalamine may reduce the risk of disease recurrence among patients who have had surgery. Recent data also suggest that mesalamine may decrease the risk of colon cancer in people with UC, but little data are yet available regarding risk reduction in patients with CD of the colon.

Mesalamine treatment is generally well tolerated by children. Unfortunately, the tablet formulations cannot be broken or chewed, and a pharmacist cannot make liquid preparations without losing the beneficial action of the medication. For children unable to swallow whole tablets or capsules, a formulation that comes in a capsule can typically be opened, and the granules can be placed in a small amount of a soft solid such as yogurt, applesauce, or pudding. Today, many doctors prefer to prescribe mesalamine rather than sulfasalazine, to avoid the potential side effects of the sulfa in sulfasalazine. Kidney injury can rarely occur with mesalamine and is more common in the elderly. Routine blood tests can help monitor for this potential side effect. Mesalamine is safe during conception and pregnancy and has no effect on male fertility. As with all medications, read the information on the 5-ASA drugs provided by the pharmacist and discuss with the health care team any questions you have.

Topical 5-ASA Medications

Topical (surface medication) 5-ASA preparations are often prescribed for people with inflammation in the lower portions of the large intestine such as the sigmoid colon and rectum (called *proctosigmoiditis* or *proctitis*). Mesalamine suppositories and enemas are associated with higher remission rates and greater clinical improvement than steroid-based topical treatments (see below for information on corticosteroids).

Topical mesalamine treatment is more effective than oral treatment when colitis is restricted to the lowest part of the colon, although combined topical and oral treatment often produces greater improvement than either treatment alone. Once in remission, patients may be instructed to continue taking not only daily oral treatment, but also topical treatment three to four times each week, to maintain remission.

Corticosteroids

Perhaps the best known of the medications used to induce remission are corticosteroids, also referred to as steroids. These drugs can rapidly bring on remission, controlling the most troubling symptoms within days or, at most, weeks. Corticosteroids work systemically—that is, throughout the body. Because these medications are effective wherever the inflammation is located in the digestive system, they are useful in treating both Crohn's disease and ulcerative colitis. Most patients achieve clinical remission with steroid treatment.

Corticosteroids do not cure IBD, however, and they have not been found to heal the lining of the intestine. These medications are for short-term use only—not only is there no long-term benefit, but a significant number of patients become steroid dependent. It is crucial that your child's doctor recommend an effective long-term medication to maintain remission without the need for steroids. Many experts do not consider a patient to be truly in remission until she is symptom-free and not taking corticosteroids.

Corticosteroids are known as much for their adverse side effects as for their positive effects. The side effects of corticosteroids increase the longer

Table 10.3
Side effects of corticosteroids

Short term

• Increased appetite	• Accelerated bone loss (weaker bones)
• Weight gain, especially in the face, upper trunk, and back	• Headache
• Stomach irritation	• Increased blood pressure
• Mood swings	• Sleeping difficulties
• Fluid retention	• Flushing
	• Acne

Long term

• Vulnerability to infections (lowered immunity)	• Drug interactions (discuss with doctor or pharmacist)
• Muscle weakness, especially around the shoulder and hip muscles	• Poor wound healing
• Elevated blood sugar	• Stretch marks
• Bone death (avascular necrosis) of the head of the thigh bone or upper arm bone	• Personality changes (irritability, psychosis, depression)
	• Acne
• Accelerated bone loss (weaker bones)	• Irregular periods
	• Delayed growth
• Cataracts	• Increased facial and body hair
• High blood pressure	• Glaucoma
	• Adrenal gland suppression

they are used. The more doses a patient takes, the greater and more serious the side effects. This is another reason patients should use these medications for only a limited time. A sudden stop of corticosteroids can also cause dangerous side effects, so patients must follow a schedule for tapering off this medication.

Doctors usually prescribe steroids at relatively high doses for a short time to bring on relief of symptoms. Once symptoms are under control, the dose is slowly reduced, and eventually the medication is stopped, usually within six or eight weeks.

The side effects associated with long-term use of corticosteroids are displayed in table 10.3. As we have learned more about steroid use over the years, recommendations for their use have changed. These changes include

- limiting the cumulative dose of corticosteroids (that is, the total amount a patient takes over time)—ideally, a child will not need to take more than one course of corticosteroids
- weaning carefully and at the right time—corticosteroids should not be stopped too quickly or all at once
- combining corticosteroids with immunomodulators or biologics to reduce the required steroid dose
- giving newer forms of corticosteroids with fewer side effects
- monitoring carefully for side effects

For moderate and severe disease, systemic corticosteroids (table 10.4) are given by mouth to a maximum of typically 40 to 60 milligrams per day (mg/day). This dose may be modified if certain medications, which affect the liver metabolism (breakdown) of corticosteroids, are taken at the same time. Drinking large amounts of grapefruit juice slows the liver's ability to break down corticosteroids, so you need to limit the amount of grapefruit juice your child drinks while taking these medications.

Corticosteroids can be given only once per day, but if your child's doctor has recommended that the steroids be given more than once per day at first, the dosage may be switched to once in the morning when an improvement is seen. Providing steroids in this way mimics the body's production of its own steroid stress hormones and helps decrease some of the drug's short-term side effects. For teenagers, the cosmetic effects of steroids (for example, weight gain or acne) are a big problem with using these medications.

Table 10.4
Pill, intravenous, and rectal forms of corticosteroids

Pill (oral)

    Prednisone, prednisolone, budesonide

Intravenous

    Methylprednisolone, hydrocortisone

Rectal (enema or suppository)

    Hydrocortisone, budesonide

If oral corticosteroids (those taken by mouth) are not having an effect, or if the patient is hospitalized, steroids are generally given intravenously (through an IV) several times during the day. If there is no response within a week, it is unlikely that there will be a response to this class of drugs. Patients who do not respond to corticosteroids are called *steroid resistant*.

Among patients who are helped by corticosteroids, oral steroid treatments continue for several weeks, and then doctors start to gradually decrease the dose. Some patients may be able to discontinue their steroids without a flare of their disease, but other patients may be classified as *steroid dependent*. That is because they will have a flare when they reduce or stop their steroid medication. Because many patients are steroid dependent, corticosteroids are commonly combined with 5-ASAs, immunomodulators, or biologics. The combination may start as soon as corticosteroids are prescribed or after it becomes clear that a patient is steroid dependent. Steroid-dependent patients require an increase in corticosteroid dose to control their symptoms again.

Corticosteroids are powerful medications that must be taken every day, exactly as prescribed. Missing doses, or decreasing the amount of steroids too quickly after taking them for several weeks, can have serious and bad effects on the body. The problem occurs because the body's adrenal glands produce natural steroid hormones. The adrenal glands will produce less of the body's natural steroids if they are taken in pill form. Once it senses that the corticosteroid levels in the bloodstream are lower, it starts producing these steroids again, very slowly.

If the person is left without any steroids in the bloodstream, many problems can develop (table 10.5). If corticosteroids are stopped suddenly, the adrenal gland will not be able to compensate quickly enough, and can leave the body without any natural steroids to handle stress. This situation can become dangerous. But with slow tapering off of oral steroids, the adrenal glands will again produce their usual level of natural steroids without long-term bad effects.

In addition to giving your child corticosteroids every day, exactly as your child's doctor prescribes, it is important to notify the doctor if a child taking steroids develops an infection, needs surgery, or is involved in a

Table 10.5
Symptoms of stopping corticosteroids too quickly after long-term use

• Nausea with or without vomiting	• Muscle pain
• Fatigue	• Fever
• Loss of appetite	• Joint pains
• Shortness of breath or difficulty in breathing	• Dizziness
• Low blood sugar	• Skin peeling
• Low blood pressure	• Fainting
• Feeling of uneasiness or general discomfort	• Irregular heartbeats

serious accident. These unusual stresses to the body may require temporary increases in the steroid treatment. Normally, the adrenal gland would be pushed to make more natural steroid under these stressful conditions. But it may not be able to do so when a person is taking corticosteroids. Finally, if a child taking corticosteroids develops an illness with vomiting and is unable to keep the medication in the stomach long enough for the medication to be absorbed, the child should go to the hospital. Doctors in the hospital may decide to start an IV, and corticosteroids will be given through that route.

Corticosteroids can cause significant irritation and even ulceration in the stomach, so your child's doctor will likely prescribe an antacid while your child is taking corticosteroids. To minimize the swollen appearance and water retention with taking steroids, your child should try to avoid salty foods such as chips, french fries, and pizza, and certainly should not add extra salt to foods.

Patients with IBD affecting the rectum and sigmoid colon (lower part of the colon) may be treated with enemas containing hydrocortisone. Only about 25 percent of the enema dose is absorbed into the bloodstream. Although patients may still experience side effects from the enemas, the side effects might be less severe.

Budesonide is a corticosteroid medication that is made with special coatings that allow it to bypass the stomach and be released slowly to target particular sections of the intestines. It offers an alternative to systemic corticosteroids for patients with IBD. Certain preparations disperse in the last part of the small intestine (ileum) and the first part of the colon (cecum) to treat CD. Other preparations are formulated to disperse more broadly in the colon to treat UC. Budesonide is also available as a foam enema, for patients with disease of the rectum and sigmoid. This form of steroid is rapidly broken down in the body after passing through the digestive tract, and therefore its side effects are greatly decreased compared with corticosteroids. Though budesonide causes fewer side effects than other corticosteroids, and the side effects are slower to develop, patients are still at risk for them. As with systemic corticosteroids, budesonide doses should decrease slowly, to prevent the development of adrenal gland problems. Unfortunately, although side effects are reduced, budesonide is not as effective as systemic corticosteroids, and there also appears to be no benefit to taking it long term to prevent disease relapse.

Antibiotics

Antibiotics play a role in the treatment of inflammatory bowel disease. Doctors often prescribe them for specific symptoms, including *perianal* (around the anus) complications from Crohn's disease. Sometimes doctors prescribe antibiotics in addition to the other medications discussed in this chapter to help bring flares under control.

Patients with IBD have a problem with the way their immune system works. Normally, the immune system prevents infections by providing protection from invading bacteria. In IBD, although no identifiable infection is present, the immune system acts inappropriately against normal bacteria that live in the intestine, attacking areas of the intestines as if an infection were present, and this leads to chronic inflammation. It is thought that antibiotics can help reduce the inflammation by changing the amount and type of bacteria in the intestines.

Antibiotics may also help treat fistulas, which are abnormal inflammatory openings from a portion of the intestine to other nearby structures, including skin, bladder, and vagina. Treatment with antibiotics against the bacteria that normally live in the bowel, along with medication directed against the inflammation of CD, may help heal fistulas. In addition, antibiotics may help patients with CD who have disease activity in their colon and around their anus.

Metronidazole and ciprofloxacin are the two most studied antibiotics in CD. Because of potential side effects of these drugs, neither should be used long term, but a course of several weeks of one or both can be useful for some patients. Another antibiotic, rifaximin, has also been helpful in adults and children with CD, especially among those who have an overgrowth of normal bacteria in the small intestine (*small intestinal bacterial overgrowth*, or SIBO) and who have resulting bloating, gas, and abdominal pain.

Although no specific bacteria or infections are known to cause IBD, *Clostridium difficile* is one particular bacterium that deserves special mention. *C. difficile* (often called *C. diff* by doctors) is a bacterium that can overgrow in the bowel, especially after a patient has been exposed to antibiotics for any reason. The toxins it makes can cause a bowel inflammation resembling the colitis of IBD and has been associated with disease flares in people with IBD. Even though the risk of this infection may be *increased* by exposure to antibiotics, *C. difficile* is initially treated with an antibiotic, such as metronidazole or vancomycin, and people with IBD flares may take these antibiotics to treat *C. difficile*.

In UC, treatment of a severe flare may include antibiotics because the damaged bowel lining can become infected as a result of the damage from the disease process and the presence of bacteria in the colon. If *C. difficile* is found in someone with UC, this infection should also be treated with antibiotics.

Immunomodulators

An immunomodulator is a drug that affects the immune system, and although all medicines used in the treatment of IBD affect the immune system, some by tradition have been labeled *immunomodulators*. Immunomodulator medications (table 10.6) are prescribed to counteract the overactive immune process in people with inflammatory bowel disease. Although some, such as methotrexate, cyclosporine, and tacrolimus, can be

Table 10.6
Immunomodulators (generic names)

Azathioprine
6-Mercaptopurine
Methotrexate
Cyclosporine
Tacrolimus

Only experienced gastroenterologists should prescribe immunomodulators.

used to induce remission, others, such as 6-mercaptopurine (6-MP) and its closely related medication, azathioprine (AZA), typically work to maintain remission in patients with IBD.

The use of immunomodulators in the treatment of IBD has greatly improved the likelihood of response, while allowing reduction or discontinuation of corticosteroid medications in children. As studies continue to monitor the long-term efficacy of these medications, doctors who treat children and adolescents have found these drugs to be important options in the therapy of pediatric IBD. In the next section, we review the role of other immunomodulating medications in the treatment of children and teens with IBD.

Reasons for Choosing Immunomodulators in Children

Although corticosteroids are effective in reducing disease activity in many children with acute UC or CD, there are clear reasons for considering immunomodulators:

- Some patients do not respond to corticosteroid treatments or become dependent on corticosteroids, and
- the potential side effects of corticosteroids, especially long term, are severe.

Azathioprine and 6-Mercaptopurine

AZA and 6-MP are currently among the best studied of the steroid-sparing immunomodulators used to treat IBD in children and teens and have been used for decades. They are similar medications that lead to the same active metabolites (breakdown products) in the body. Many pediatric gastroenterologists include one of these drugs in the initial treatment of children with newly diagnosed moderate to severe Crohn's disease or ulcerative colitis as they have been shown to increase corticosteroid-free periods, maintain remission, and decrease the frequency of relapses.

AZA and 6-MP are given by mouth, and deciding on the best dose in individual patients depends on how well they metabolize the drug. Before starting AZA or 6-MP, your child's doctor will do a blood test to check an enzyme (a protein) in your child's body that will help decide whether your child can break down the drug appropriately. Once your child is taking AZA or 6-MP, a different blood test can be done periodically to measure blood levels of an important metabolite called 6-thioguanine (6-TG), which is the active anti-inflammatory ingredient of these drugs. This enables doctors to adjust the dose to a specific target range known to be therapeutic. Furthermore, other metabolites that increase the risk of elevated liver enzymes can also be monitored and the dosage adjusted or the drug discontinued if necessary.

Some children who receive these drugs are not able to continue treatment because of either a serious reaction to the medication (such as pancreatitis) or intolerance (nausea, abdominal pain, or repeat infections). These medications can also suppress production of cells in the bone marrow, causing a decrease in white blood cells or temporary elevations in liver enzymes. AZA and 6-MP may also slightly increase a person's risk of developing a future cancer (such as lymphoma). Children need to be up to date on all immunizations before starting AZA or 6-MP because no one should receive live-virus vaccines while taking these drugs. Seek medical attention if your child develops high fever, is exposed to chicken pox (if not previously infected with this virus), or shows other signs and symptoms of potentially serious infectious illnesses.

Methotrexate

Some children cannot tolerate AZA or 6-MP. For these children, as well as for those who are corticosteroid dependent, additional drug choices are necessary. Based in part on the results of adult studies, pediatric gastroenterologists may choose instead to use methotrexate (MTX), which is given once a week as an injection under the skin or as a once weekly oral dose. Doctors may decide it's best to start MTX as injection because of concerns that the oral form may not be absorbed as well during periods of intestinal inflammation. Patients who are responding well to MTX may be able to switch to the oral form at a later time. This drug's effectiveness is well established in adult CD, and the experience in using it in children has been similar. It has not been well studied in patients with UC.

Much of the information about the safety of MTX in children comes from long-term experience in children with juvenile idiopathic arthritis who receive MTX. Just as with AZA and 6-MP, safety monitoring is important with those taking MTX, including regular reviews of complete blood count and liver enzyme tests. A child with acute or chronic liver disease should typically not receive MTX. The possible development of liver scarring (fibrosis or cirrhosis) is a concern long-term use and seems to be related to an excessive cumulative dose, but this type of scarring is very rarely seen in children. Finally, while methotrexate is generally safe and well tolerated, it can harm a developing fetus at the time the medication is taken, and therefore *should not be used by any female who might become pregnant* while on the medication.

Cyclosporine and Tacrolimus

Use of cyclosporine (also called cyclosporine-A) or tacrolimus (also called FK506) should be considered only in patients with severe cases of ulcerative colitis or Crohn's disease that do not respond to traditional medications. Both medications are strong immunosuppressants—that is, they significantly lower a person's immunity. Whether the risks of harsh potential side effects of these medications outweigh their benefits is still uncertain. Most often, these medications are used as a "bridge" to other therapies, including surgery, because they are not as effective in the long term. Several small studies in adults found a possible short-term benefit to intravenous cyclosporine treatment for patients with severe UC (disease that did not respond to other treatments). With or without the addition of steroids, cyclosporine treatment decreased the need for emergency removal of the colon (colectomy). When treatment with this drug stops, though, the relapse rate is very high. If cyclosporine is used, it should be prescribed with the understanding that colectomy most likely will still be necessary within a year.

No studies have evaluated cyclosporine in children with severe CD. Studies in adults have shown that low doses do not induce or maintain remission in patients with long-term active CD. High-dose cyclosporine may help achieve remission, but high doses are associated with serious and harmful effects.

Cyclosporine can cause toxicity to the kidneys, high blood pressure, nervous-system side effects, and nausea and vomiting. Swelling of the gums and increased hair growth usually happen as well. *Pneumocystis* pneumonia, an unusual infection seen only in immunosuppressed individuals, may develop during cyclosporine treatment. Therefore, doctors normally prescribe treatment with antibiotics against *Pneumocystis* when treating patients with cyclosporine. Post-transplant lymphoproliferative disease (which may be complicated by lymphoma) is a rare complication of cyclosporine treatments and is reported primarily in patients who have undergone solid organ transplants.

Tacrolimus, which is taken only by mouth, is a stronger immunosuppressive medication than cyclosporine. It is also more reliably absorbed from the intestine into the bloodstream. In a few studies of tacrolimus treatment in children, the majority of patients with steroid-resistant severe colitis achieved short-term remission, and approximately half were in remission one year later. No long-term data on these patients are available.

Similar to cyclosporine, tacrolimus can cause kidney toxicity, high blood pressure, nervous-system side effects, and nausea and vomiting, and it can increase the risk of acquiring *Pneumocystis* pneumonia. As with cyclosporine, doctors normally prescribe treatment with antibiotics against *Pneumocystis* when treating patients with tacrolimus. Post-transplant lymphoproliferative disease (which may be complicated by lymphoma) is also a rare complication of tacrolimus treatments and again is reported primarily in patients who have undergone solid organ transplants.

Biologics

A biologic medication is different from most drugs available on the market. Most drugs are smaller molecules with very well-known structures and are made using a chemical process that can be easily replicated. Biologics are made in a living system, such as in microorganisms or plant or animal cells. Most biologics are large and complex molecules or combinations of molecules. They are produced by biotechnology methods and other innovative technologies.

Anti-tumor Necrosis Factor-Alpha Therapy

Anti-TNFα medications (table 10.7) have greatly influenced the course of illness in many children and adolescents with difficult-to-control IBD. Reported benefits include

- disease remission
- healing of fistulas
- reduction and discontinuation of corticosteroids
- improved growth

Anti-TNFα medicines include infliximab, adalimumab, certolizumab, and golimumab. Some have been approved by regulatory agencies such as the Food and Drug Administration (FDA) for treating children with Crohn's disease and ulcerative colitis. These medications are manufactured proteins, called antibodies, that interfere with another protein—tumor necrosis factor-alpha (TNFα), which plays a key role in the inflammatory process in IBD. Anti-TNFα medicines can be extremely effective in bringing CD and UC into quick steroid-free remission, and they have dra-

Table 10.7
Anti-TNFα medications

Infliximab
Adalimumab
Certolizumab
Golimumab

Only experienced gastroenterologists should prescribe biologic agents.

matically changed the management of IBD since the FDA approved the first anti-TNFα, infliximab, in 1998. They are systemic medications (active throughout the body), given either intravenously or by injection under the skin. Since these biologics can have a dramatic response, doctors use them typically for patients with moderate to severe CD or UC, including those who are not responding to corticosteroids or immunomodulators.

A significant number of children who receive anti-TNFα medications will improve with these treatments, even if they have not responded to prior therapies. Infliximab and adalimumab have been evaluated in clinical trials specifically in children—the REACH and IMAGINE trials. These studies demonstrated to the public and to the FDA that the medications were safe and very effective for treating IBD in children.

Children who are being treated with infliximab typically receive three IV doses in the first six weeks to induce remission, then scheduled doses about every two months to maintain remission. Children receiving adalimumab typically receive doses via injection under the skin about every two weeks. The first two adalimumab injections are meant to induce remission and are often larger doses than the doses that follow about every two weeks. Depending on how effective the medication is, your child's physician may choose to vary the dose or interval. Response to these medications is fairly prompt, though, and if your child does not respond in the first three months, other treatments may need to be considered or further evaluations performed to ensure that your child's symptoms are due to his IBD.

Most children tolerate infliximab and adalimumab very well. The side effects of infliximab may be acute (occurring during or within a few hours after the infusion), or delayed (up to seven days after the infusion). Shortness of breath or rash can occur in a small percentage of children during the infusion. More severe acute reactions are rare, but they can include shortness of breath or rash, a drop in blood pressure, swelling or wheezing, and sometimes extensive redness or hives all over the body. Delayed reactions include fever, joint pains or swelling (arthritis), headache, and malaise (general ill feeling). If a patient has an infusion reaction, the infusion is typically discontinued and the patient is evaluated. If the reactions are mild, the infusion may be restarted at the same rate or at a slower rate. Infusion reactions may be treated with medications such as one or more doses of corticosteroids. Other medicines may be required as needed based on the instructions of your child's doctor to the infusion team. Similarly, patients taking adalimumab may experience side effects during or within hours of their injection, including injection-site pain, redness, itching, or swelling. Side effects days after an injection may include headache or upper respiratory infections. Again, if your child has any of these side effects, discuss them with your child's doctor.

The dramatic success of infliximab and adalimumab has led to the development of other anti-TNFα medications. For example, certolizumab and golimumab are injectable biologics also used in the treatment of IBD. Although they have not yet received similar approval by the FDA for use in children, the clinical experience for these newer anti-TNFαs is increasing and they may be beneficial for children who have developed an allergic reaction to infliximab or adalimumab or whose disease has lost response to those medications.

Deciding whether to prescribe an anti-TNFα medication for a child with IBD can sometimes be a difficult decision. Discussions between the patient, parents, and health care team are essential in these situations. As with all medications, discussing a therapy's pros and cons is important. In this conversation, keep in mind that IBD itself can be quite serious and that treatment is what will help your child regain good health and thrive. During discussions of medication risk, your child's doctor should speak to you about what might happen to your child without treatment, or with suboptimal treatment.

Pivotal trials in adults with IBD using combinations of immunomodulators (AZA, 6-MP, or MTX) and anti-TNFα biologic therapies have been translated to the care of children with IBD. A combination of the two may often be more effective than using one or the other on its own. The greater effectiveness of the combination may happen for several reasons. First, the body tends to react to foreign proteins like anti-TNFα medications, forming its own antibodies against the biologics. These antibodies can remove the drug quickly from circulation and may be responsible for infusion reactions, such as rash, swelling, and wheezing, that patients sometimes encounter. Theoretically, using an immunomodulator with a biologic may prevent the body from developing antibodies against anti-TNFα drugs. In addition, because immunomodulators and biologics may be effective on their own, in combination they may have a "synergistic" effect, acting more powerfully than when they are used alone.

Although anti-TNFα medications have been well studied in adults and children with IBD, these drugs are still relatively new, and questions about their use remain. The FDA has mandated that companies producing these medications maintain long-term safety registries of patients who take them. The information gathered so far on their safety indicates that they are, in general, safe; however, we need to continue monitoring the patients who receive them to learn more about any potential long-term side effects. Very rare but serious complications of anti-TNFα therapy have been reported. These include increased risk of infections such as tuberculosis, invasive fungal infections, and herpetic skin infections. Patients receiving anti-TNFα therapy should not receive live vaccines because the therapy may allow the viral products in these vaccines to cause significant illness. Although the concern for cancers such as lymphoma has been raised with anti-TNFα therapy, recent data suggest that when compared to the general population of children, anti-TNFα medicines alone do not increase the risk of cancers in children receiving these medications. Nonetheless, patients (especially young men) on long-term combination therapy of an anti-TNFα with the immunomodulators AZA or 6-MP (but not MTX) may be at increased risk of developing a particularly aggressive type of cancer, called *hepatosplenic T-cell lymphoma* (HSTCL). Doctors were certainly aware that this cancer could occur in a person without IBD, but since the year 2000, among the millions of patients who have been exposed to anti-TNFα medicines, several dozen patients, mostly males in their late teens or early twenties who were taking an anti-TNFα with either AZA or 6-MP, were diagnosed with this cancer. Although very rare, concern about HSTCL has led to changes in how pediatric gastroenterologists treat children with IBD. When 6-MP or AZA are prescribed in combination with anti-TNFα medications, doctors tend to limit the use of these immunomodulators to a shorter period, such as the first six months of therapy. Alternatively, physicians use methotrexate in combination with anti-TNFα medications, because the same cancer concerns have not as yet been observed with this particular combination of immunomodulator and anti-TNFα therapy.

Anti-Adhesion Medicines

Newer treatments beyond anti-TNFα medicines have continued to build on the success of biologics. A potential disadvantage of a biologic is that with repeated treatments, the immune system may begin to recognize this foreign protein and develop antibodies against the drug, which decreases its effectiveness and increases its side effects. Manufacturers of anti-TNFα biologics have tried to make the proteins as humanlike as possible to avoid the development of anti-drug proteins, but the antibodies still develop and may decrease a person's ability to tolerate multiple anti-TNFα medications. Thus biologics that help calm down the immune system in other ways besides attacking the TNFα protein have been developed.

A promising class of biologics is the *anti-adhesion* medications, also called *selective adhesion molecule inhibitors*. These medications work by an entirely different mechanism than that of the anti-TNFα medications. They interfere with the ability of certain immune cells, called white blood cells, to adhere (attach) to the cells lining blood vessels so that the white blood cells cannot exit the bloodstream and enter the intestinal tissue. (These white blood cells are involved in initiating the inflammation of IBD.) Interrupting this process may reduce the inflammation and improve symptoms of the disease. The first demonstration that this type of approach could be effective was with the drug natalizumab. This antibody binds to an immune cell protein called alpha-4 integrin. Alpha-4 integrin is a protein that immune cells use to travel to both the intestine and the brain for surveillance against foreign invaders. Natalizumab is approved by the FDA to treat resistant Crohn's disease in adults, and there is some evidence that this drug may help children as well. The biggest concern about natalizumab, however, is that because it is not very selective, and because it keeps immune cells from carrying out important surveillance in the brain, it appears to increase the risk of developing progressive multifocal leukoencephalopathy, a rare and often fatal viral infection of the central nervous system.

To overcome this safety concern, scientists developed a more selective drug that blocks immune cells from entering the intestine but allows them to do their important work in the brain. This drug, called vedolizumab, blocks the protein alpha-4/beta-7 integrin, which is specific for the white blood cells traveling to the intestine. Vedolizumab is FDA approved to treat moderate to severe CD or UC in adults. It seems to be more effective in UC than CD, but patients with CD who have primarily colonic inflammation may benefit from vedolizumab. Very few studies are available in children, although the pediatric experience is increasing and like adults, vedolizumab appears to help children with UC or colonic CD.

Similar to infliximab, vedolizumab is given as three IV doses in the first six weeks, then scheduled doses are given about every two months. Unlike infliximab and the other anti-TNFα medicines, vedolizumab's full effect may not be noted until the patient has been receiving it for twelve to fourteen weeks. This means that other medicines, such as 5-ASAs or corticosteroids, may be required to help induce remission while waiting for vedolizumab to have its full effect. Similar to what happens with the anti-TNFα medicines, the frequency of dosing may be changed by your child's doctor based on your child's clinical response or information about drug levels in the bloodstream.

Vedolizumab appears to be well tolerated. Some people have headaches and very few get infusion reactions. Long-term studies are limited, since this medication was only FDA approved in 2014, but as of now, there appears to be no significant increase in the risk of serious infections or cancer.

Newer Drugs and Others on the Horizon

Just as TNFα is a key protein involved in the inflammatory pathway that leads to IBD, many other proteins (cytokines) also participate in the inflammatory process. For example, the cytokines named IL-12 and IL-23 also have central roles in driving the inflammatory response in IBD by stimulating particular white blood cells called T helper 1 (Th1) and T helper 17 (Th17) cells. Ustekinumab, a biologic antibody that targets IL-12 and IL-23, was approved for the treatment of moderate to severe Crohn's disease in adults in 2016. The benefits of this medication were noted as early as a few weeks from the start of therapy, suggesting that ustekinumab is helpful for inducing remission as well as keeping symptoms under control over a longer period. Ustekinumab is given by an infusion at the beginning and then an injection under the skin about every two months. The data are still sparse for its use in children but hopefully will increase in the near future. Although no serious infection, cancer, or other concerning side effects have been noted, longer safety monitoring is required.

While there are multiple biologic therapies for IBD, such as etrolizumab, brazikumab, and risankizumab, in current clinical trials, other drugs that are not biologics are still being developed to target the inflammatory pathways that lead to IBD. As mentioned earlier in this chapter, while biologics are large, complex drugs that are produced in living cell cultures, *small molecule* medications are more simple and are produced by a chemical process. Most familiar medicines on the market, such as aspirin or the acid blocker omeprazole, are small molecule drugs. For IBD, some small molecule medications show early promise in treating adults. These include tofacitinib, a pill that is undergoing adult trials for moderately to severely active UC, and mongersen, also a pill, with early good results in patients with CD. Dozens of other drugs are making their way through the research pipeline for IBD treatment, so the future remains hopeful that more medications that are safe and have even fewer side effects will soon be available to treat both CD and UC.

Biosimilars

Patents for many of the early biologics such as infliximab and adalimumab are beginning to expire. This has resulted in the development of biosimilars with the potential for significant savings for health care insurers and patients. A *biosimilar* is a biologic medicine that is similar to another biologic medicine (called the *originator* or *innovator*) that has already been authorized for use. A biosimilar is not the same thing as a generic version of a drug. Generic drugs are pretty much exact copies of brand-name drugs, but since biologics are huge, complex proteins grown

in living systems, it is not possible to absolutely replicate this process—
therefore the drug that is made is "similar" but not an exact copy of the
original. A biosimilar is approved if manufacturers have been able to show
that the product has no clinically meaningful differences in terms of safety
and effectiveness from the originator reference product. Biosimilars also
need to have the same mechanisms of action, route of administration, and
dosage form and strength as the originator drug. Biosimilars have been
used in Europe since about 2005, but the first two biosimilars to infliximab and adalimumab were approved in the United States by the FDA in
2016. We will learn more about these products and have a better idea
whether they help reduce health care costs in the United States when
they become more widely available in the U.S. market.

Nutritional Therapy

The role of nutrition as supplemental therapy for growth and sexual development is discussed in greater detail in chapter 13. In this chapter we
discuss nutrition as a primary therapy to induce remission in patients with
Crohn's disease. Studies have shown that a particular form of nutrition,
called *exclusive enteral nutrition* (EEN), can be as effective as corticosteroids in inducing remission. Other studies have shown that the only therapy for CD, besides anti-TNFα drugs, known to positively affect a child's
skeletal growth is EEN.

In nutritional therapy, specialized formulas are used to make sure patients are receiving all the nutrients—vitamins and minerals—they need
for healing and growth. We know that on average, children with CD may
require up to 50 percent more calories than their peers. Your child's physician can calculate a goal number of calories each day, and these can be
provided as primary nutritional therapy.

The formulas can be taken orally, but if a child does not like the taste, or
gets bored with the taste, a nasogastric (NG) tube can be passed through her
nose into her stomach to administer the formula. Children and teens are often taught how to place their own NG tubes at night and remove them each
morning if they do not want to attend school with the NG tube in place.

Because children with CD may be uncomfortable initially with large volumes of calories delivered quickly, the feeding amounts are slowly increased over the first several days of the therapy until the goal is reached. During the treatment period, which in most cases is six to eight weeks, this formula may be the primary food that your child will receive. In general, physicians recommend that for these first six to eight weeks, 80 to 90 percent of calories be delivered by special formulas. That means 10 to 20 percent of your child's daily calories can be consumed as foods by mouth. Often your child's doctor or dietician will give you recommendations on what types of foods should make up that 10 to 20 percent. When your child is in remission, the tube feeds may be decreased and normal food reintroduced in larger quantities.

We do not understand exactly why this nutritional therapy is so effective at inducing remission. In part, however, EEN may be changing the composition of the bacteria that inhabit the intestine, making them less likely to cause the immune system to overreact. By removing most regular foods from your child's diet, you may also be removing additives or other products within the food system that may eventually be identified as promoting intestinal inflammation. If EEN is effective in inducing remission, children may eventually tolerate more of their calories delivered by table foods. But IBD is more likely to flare when the feedings are stopped completely, so to maintain remission, medical therapy is often used to help manage the IBD.

Pediatric IBD Research

Pediatric IBD doctors have been at the forefront of research, advancing the state of the art of science into fields such as genetics and the microbiome. Pediatric research network projects sponsored by the Crohn's and Colitis Foundation and the National Institutes of Health (NIH) have generated volumes of important new discoveries. For example, the RISK and PROTECT projects have studied thousands of newly diagnosed children with CD or UC to determine factors that contribute to these complicated conditions. The important insights pediatric gastroenterologists have gathered identify possible new targets for drugs and teach physicians when it is most appropriate to prescribe the medications we have available.

Since the groundbreaking work that showed the usefulness of infliximab in IBD, the pipeline of biologics and other medications that have entered human clinical trials has picked up at a more rapid pace than ever before. IBD clinical trials are usually done first in adults, and then some are done in children. Advocacy for pediatric IBD, delivered in part by the North American Society for Pediatric Gastroenterology, Hepatology and Nutrition (NASPGHAN) and by the Crohn's and Colitis Foundation, has led to a required focus on children during the drug approval process at the U.S. federal level. Public forums sponsored by the FDA brought into focus the pediatric IBD treating physicians' concerns about a lag in pediatric approvals and the need to use new drugs *off label* (for uses not FDA approved). Although there may be a significant pediatric experience with a medication, if it is not FDA approved for use in children, insurers can decide to not cover its costs or deny its use in a child, even if the patient's doctor believes it is the best medicine to use for that child's IBD.

Summary of Induction and Remission Treatment

Treatment for IBD is typically focused on inducing remission and then maintaining it. Various combinations of medications can be used in this process, including 5-aminosalicylates, corticosteroids, immunomodulators, antibiotics, and biologic therapies. At the moment there is no "standard of care" regarding which medications should be used in particular cases or clinical scenarios. For example, a 5-ASA may be the best option for your child if she has mild symptoms of IBD, whereas a biologic agent may make more sense for a child with more significant symptoms. New treatments for children and teens with IBD continue to be developed, providing additional options for patients with nonresponsive disease, often leading to reduced use, or discontinuation, of corticosteroids. As new medications become available, special considerations in children, such as bone abnormalities, growth, infection risks, and differences in drug breakdown, will need to be studied. Large pediatric studies now under way are trying to identify how we can best predict, at the time of diagnosis, which medicine and treatment pathway is ideal for a particular patient. We hope that all the research currently being done will enable doctors to use the best therapy at the right time for a particular child.

Therapy for Crohn's disease and ulcerative colitis is changing rapidly, and it can be challenging for a family to weigh the risks and benefits of various treatments. But this is also an exciting time filled with promise for better therapies for IBD. Patients and families should ask as many questions as necessary to become comfortable with IBD treatment options. In response, health care professionals should provide information in clear language. Teaching materials such as pamphlets, books, and articles, as well as contact with support groups, are often very helpful. In this age of online information, each family should be encouraged to get as much information as possible from the child's health care team, rather than from the Internet. Online information often does not relate to children and is not always accurate. Patient forums tend to trumpet miraculous treatments that work for few and select situations, or relate poor experiences with therapies that apply to individual circumstances. You can rely on information from major organizations such as NASPGHAN, the Crohn's and Colitis Foundation, the Centers for Disease Control and Prevention (CDC), and NIH, but again, information about disease and treatment in adults may not be applicable in children. That is why it is important to have ongoing discussions with your child's IBD doctor whenever you have any questions about your child's current therapy or other therapies that you hear about.

回 11

Surgery

Surgery is an important part of treatment for both Crohn's disease and ulcerative colitis. It is not necessarily a last resort with IBD as it is with other conditions. Some people may benefit from surgery early in the treatment of their disease. In fact, doctors may recommend early surgical treatment along with medications, and many patients with IBD will require some type of surgery during the course of their illness.

Who Needs Surgery?

Although deciding whether to perform surgery for IBD often carries with it a great deal of worry, in certain situations, the decision to operate is made relatively easily. These situations include cases of uncontrollable bleeding, perforations (holes in the intestine), obstruction (complete blockage), and intestinal cancer. In such *emergent* (urgent) situations, the type of intestinal disease (CD or UC) is not an important consideration, because surgery is the only helpful approach to treatment. When surgery is to be performed *electively* (by choice), however, deciding to undergo an operation, and determining when it should be performed, is more difficult.

The goals of IBD treatment are

to heal the lining of the intestine,
to ease or stop symptoms,
to improve general health, and
to improve growth, sexual development, and dietary condition.

The purpose of surgery is to reach these goals when medication treatment has failed or become too toxic, while trying to save as much of the intestine as possible. The decision about whether surgery is necessary is made based on medical history and physical exam (chapter 6), imaging studies (chapter 8), and endoscopic exams (chapter 9).

Patients and their families should discuss surgery, including the potential advantages and disadvantages, with the entire medical team. This team usually includes many specialists, such as a pediatric gastroenterologist, an IBD surgeon, a nurse practitioner, a nutritionist, and a psychologist. All treatment options should be discussed thoroughly. Only in this way can everyone feel confident that the best decision is being made about the next step in treatment.

When it comes to choosing a surgeon, it is important to look for someone experienced and familiar with the special features of caring for children and adolescents with IBD. The surgeon should also employ state-of-the-art advances in the field of IBD surgery.

Support organizations can provide essential information on quality of life after surgery. It is also helpful for children who are facing surgery to talk to other children who have had similar operations done. In addition, planning for surgery, making home care arrangements, and taking care of health insurance issues will free you to concentrate on providing the support your child needs.

General Terms

There are two main surgical approaches to IBD surgery: laparotomy and laparoscopy. *Laparotomy*, or open surgery, is the method requiring only one abdominal incision (cut), but it is a somewhat long cut. An alternative method, called *laparoscopy*, makes use of instruments that are inserted into the abdomen through several small openings. Laparoscopy leaves multiple very small scars.

Laparoscopic surgery may be somewhat more difficult to do and should be performed only by a surgeon experienced with the technique. If done by a skilled surgeon, laparoscopy allows for an easier and faster recovery. The surgeon ultimately makes the final decision about which type of procedure to use. Sometimes it is necessary to change procedures in the operating room, even when a different surgical procedure was planned, depending on the situation encountered.

The types of surgical procedures vary depending on the type of IBD and the reason for surgery. In this chapter, we first review the reasons for surgery and the procedures used for ulcerative colitis. We then describe the different surgical treatments for Crohn's disease.

Surgery for Ulcerative Colitis

Table 11.1 lists the most common reasons for having urgent surgery and for considering surgery for ulcerative colitis. The goal of surgical treatment for UC is to cure the disease. Such surgery involves removing the large intestine, however, and is therefore not undertaken lightly. Occasionally, patients and doctors encounter surgical complications, even in the days following an operation. In addition, these surgical procedures often require changes in lifestyle. The type of surgery done depends on the reasons for the operation. Each surgery is tailored to the patient, depending on her medical history and test results.

Before describing the surgical procedures for UC, we need to briefly review stomas, appliances, and their care.

The word *stoma* originates from the Greek word for "mouth." A surgeon creates a stoma by bringing an inch or two of intestine out through the skin to the abdominal (belly) wall. The stoma opens to the outside of

---

Table 11.1
Reasons for surgery to treat ulcerative colitis

Urgent
- uncontrolled bleeding
- a hole in the intestine (perforation)
- intestinal obstruction (blockage)
- extreme swelling of the colon (toxic megacolon)
- cancer of the large intestine (colon cancer)

Optional
- poor response to medication

the body. The name of the stoma depends on which part of the intestine is brought out to the skin. For example, the stoma is a *colostomy* if part of the colon (large intestine) is brought out to the skin; an *ileostomy* means the ileum, or end of the small intestine, is brought out; and so on. There are traditionally several types of stomas, such as Kock pouch and Brooke ileostomy, among others.

In the most common type of stoma, called a Brooke ileostomy, or colostomy, the end of a loop of intestine is brought out through an opening in the abdomen, folded on itself to form a stoma, and sutured to the skin. The opening is approximately the size of a quarter, and the intestine's contents, which are usually pasty in consistency, collect in an *appliance* (a bag that is attached to the skin with adhesive). The bag must be emptied several times a day and changed every few days (figure 11.1).

The vast majority of patients (95 percent) are able to lead normal lives with a stoma, including attending school regularly, participating in sports, and taking part in most normal activities of daily life. The site of the stoma must be chosen carefully so that it is located on a flat skin sur-

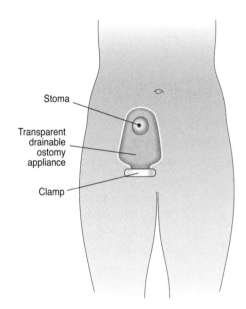

Figure 11.1. An ostomy appliance. Patients who undergo removal of the colon (because of IBD-related colitis) may require a temporary or permanent ostomy. An external ileostomy enables intestinal contents to empty into a small, discreet plastic sack that can be periodically emptied into a toilet.

Stoma

Transparent drainable ostomy appliance

Clamp

face away from creases, bony areas, and previous scars. The preferred site will locate the bag in an area where intestinal movements can easily drain into it and where emptying the bag is easy. The stoma must be positioned so that clothes fit well, sitting is comfortable, and, when possible, the bag is concealed.

An enterostomal specialist is an important member of the surgical team. Often, prior to surgery, this *stoma nurse* will mark the optimal site of an ostomy so it meets the criteria described above. He can provide advice about the appropriate type of stoma appliance and can work with the patient to troubleshoot any complications that occur (infection, leakage, and so on).

Types of Surgical Procedures for Ulcerative Colitis

Proctocolectomy with End-Ileostomy

In proctocolectomy with end-ileostomy, the entire large intestine is removed, and the end of the small intestine is brought out as a stoma. This is the least popular type of surgery since it requires a permanent appliance on the abdomen. The procedure is rarely performed now in patients with UC, and least often in children and adolescents. Occasionally, however, this surgery is necessary if the procedure called *total colectomy and ileal pouch-anal anastomosis* (IPAA) has failed.

Total Colectomy with Ileal Pouch–Anal Anastomosis

In IPAA surgery, the large intestine is removed and a pelvic "pouch" (*J pouch*, or *internal reservoir*) is created from the end of the small intestine to serve as the new rectum. The reservoir is able to hold stool. It is connected to the anus (the opening through which stool comes out of the body), allowing normal defecation (figure 11.2) at the time of the patient's choosing. This is the most popular choice for colectomy (removal of the colon) to treat UC. It can be performed in several ways.

One-stage operation is a surgical option for a minority (approximately 10 percent) of patients, and it is not always appropriate for patients with IBD (except in special situations). In this procedure, removal of the large

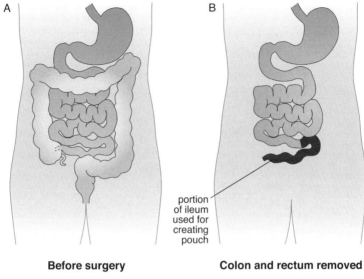

A

Before surgery

B

portion
of ileum
used for
creating
pouch

Colon and rectum removed

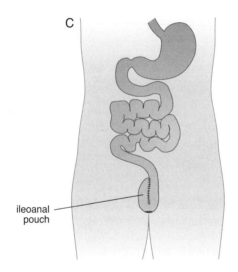

C

ileoanal
pouch

Ileoanal pouch formed

Figure 11.2. Colectomy with ileal pouch–anal anastomosis (IPAA). Most patients with ulcerative colitis who undergo colon removal do not require a permanent ileostomy. Instead, a temporary ostomy is created. In subsequent procedures, a portion of the ileum (B) is folded back on itself and pulled down to the anal region (C). Assuming this J pouch (ileoanal pouch) can be successfully created, the ileostomy can be closed and a patient can empty intestinal contents through the anus.

intestine, creation of a small intestine pouch, and connection of the pouch to the anus are done in one operation. The advantage of this method is that it does not require additional surgeries or a temporary stoma. If the intestine is inflamed at the time of this operation, however, there is a risk of poor healing, which can lead to problems.

Two-stage operation is a procedure involving removal of the large intestine, creation of the small intestine pouch, and connection to the anus. A temporary stoma on the abdomen is created and kept in place for a few months. The temporary stoma diverts movement of feces from the intestine away from the anus, so no stool passes through the anus. The stoma allows the internal pouch to heal well before stool passes through it. After two or three months, the stoma is closed and the ends of the intestine are reconnected. Once the intestine is reconnected, stool passes through the anus normally, and the stoma is no longer needed.

The three-stage operation involves first removing the colon and performing the ileostomy (opening in the abdomen). Later, after the patient recovers, the small intestine pouch is formed in a second operation, but the ileostomy remains. Finally, after more time for complete healing, the ileostomy is removed and the intestine is connected to the anus. Three-stage procedures are used when a patient has major intestinal inflammation at the time of the surgery.

After complete recovery from a total colectomy with IPAA, regardless of the number of stages, a person usually has an average of six bowel movements a day. To decrease the frequency of bowel movements, patients often receive treatments to train the small intestine pouch to store liquid stool. Additional dietary fiber and medications can help decrease the number of bowel movements. The medications slow the movement of waste through the intestine. Patients learn to stop eating several hours prior to sleep but may have to wake at night to have a bowel movement.

About 60 percent of patients who have this surgery will experience an episode of some inflammation of the pouch (a condition known as *pouchitis*) at some point after the surgery, usually within the first year. This inflammation is thought to be due to a change in the kinds of bacteria that live in that portion of the intestine, and it often resolves with a short course of antibiotics. Pouchitis episodes can occur a few times each year, but the frequency of these episodes usually decreases as time passes. Eventually, pouchitis may stop completely or occur only now and then. Chronic pouchitis, which does not go away, occurs in only a small number of patients.

Other complications after surgery include pouch leaks, fistula formation (an abnormal opening between the pouch and nearby organs), incontinence (not making it to the bathroom in time), and obstruction (blockage). Blockage may happen as a result of narrowing at the site where the pouch connects to the anus.

After surgery, as many as 1 out of 10 patients who were diagnosed with UC are later diagnosed with CD, despite all early evidence consistent with a UC diagnosis. These patients tend to have more complications after surgery. In a very small number of these patients, the ileal pouch may need to be removed and the ileostomy re-created.

Total Colectomy with Ileorectal Anastomosis

In total colectomy with ileorectal anastomosis, most of the large intestine is removed, and a straight connection is made between the end of the small intestine and the rectum (the lowermost part of the large intestine), without creating a pelvic pouch. This procedure is rarely used, since a part of the diseased large intestine is left behind after surgery. Some people believe that quality of life may be somewhat better with this procedure than after a pouch operation, because patients can have fewer bowel movements. Yet, the risk of ongoing inflammation, and the possible development of cancer in the remaining segment of the large intestine, makes this surgery less desirable. Colectomy can lead to decreased fertility (difficulties becoming pregnant) in females, often because of scarring in the pelvis that blocks the fallopian tubes, so issues of fertility should be thoroughly discussed beforehand if this is a concern.

Surgery for Crohn's Disease

The most common reasons for having surgery, whether urgently or electively, to treat CD are summarized in table 11.2. Choosing to have elective surgery can be particularly difficult for patients with CD. In UC, surgery cures the disease. But surgery for CD does not cure the illness. In fact, there is a real chance that the disease will return at some point after surgery and that the person might need more operations. Nevertheless, elective surgery is still the correct decision for a child with CD in several situations, as described below. Each case is followed by a description of the most appropriate surgery in each set of circumstances.

Scenario 1

A 15-year-old girl has had Crohn's disease for three years. Tests showed that the disease is most severe in the last portion of the small intestine. At first, the disease disappeared after steroid treatment, but every time the treatment stopped, the symptoms returned, usually abdominal pain and bloating, sometimes with diarrhea. The symptoms are often worst after eating, and to avoid symptoms, the girl has started to limit the amount that she eats. As a result, she has become malnourished—her body is not getting the food it needs to grow and stay healthy and strong.

Treatment with an immunomodulator was not effective in allowing her to stop steroid treatments and remain well. As a result, she now needs regular intravenous infusions of an anti-TNFα medication (see chapter 10). After a year of treatments with this medication, the symptoms are coming

---

Table 11.2
Reasons for surgery to treat Crohn's disease

Urgent
- uncontrolled bleeding
- obstruction (blockage)
- perforation (hole)
- abscess (infections) or fistulizing disease (when Crohn's disease causes abnormal openings between organs)

Optional
- failure of medication treatment
- stricture (narrowing in the intestine)
- perianal disease (swelling and sores around the anus)

---

back, and the girl is beginning to lose weight again. Follow-up tests show the same localized area of inflammation with some narrowing of the intestine. She is underweight and short for her age and is just starting to show signs of puberty now.

Why Surgery Might Be Right for This Adolescent

Several factors might make surgery the right choice for this girl. First, her disease has been resistant to treatment with several different medicines. Although steroids can control some of the symptoms, research shows that steroids are unlikely to bring on healing. Furthermore, steroids have many negative side effects that become increasingly undesirable the longer they are used.

A second point in favor of surgery is that the disease appears to be located in one particular area of the small intestine. This makes it unlikely that a large portion of the intestine will need to be removed.

Finally, it is critical that the child is just about to enter puberty. Puberty in this adolescent girl is already somewhat delayed at this point, and if she has continued active disease throughout this important time of growth and development, she may have permanent growth problems.

Intestinal surgery for CD in children generally involves removing the least amount of intestine possible, but enough to take care of the intestine that is clearly diseased (figure 11.3). This operation can be performed as a traditional "open" procedure, where a single cut is made in the abdominal wall, followed by examination of the intestine and removal of the diseased segment(s). The surgery can also be done as a laparoscopic procedure, where the intestine is removed using small tools inserted into the abdomen through several small incisions. Laparoscopic surgery for CD is used more and more often because recovery is faster and there is less pain after surgery. In complicated cases, though, it may be safer to perform the surgery open.

Scenario 2

A 12-year-old child has had Crohn's disease for five years. He was treated with steroids after diagnosis. Steroids were not needed again after the first

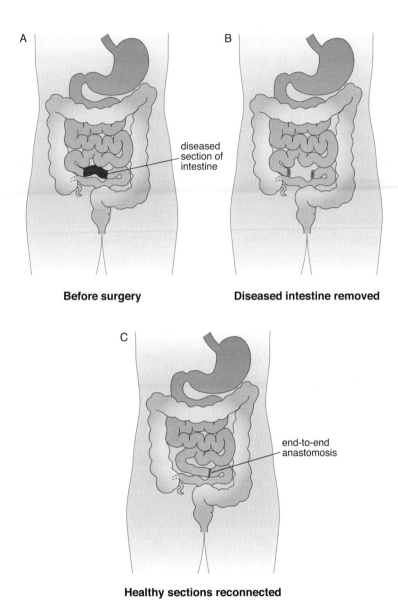

A

diseased section of intestine

Before surgery

B

Diseased intestine removed

C

end-to-end anastomosis

Healthy sections reconnected

Figure 11.3. Bowel resection and end-to-end anastomosis. In Crohn's disease, a small region of bowel sometimes needs to be removed because of inflammation, perforation, or narrowing. In most cases, the diseased section is removed, and the two healthy sections are reconnected. Assuming the amount of bowel removed is small, intestinal function is usually normal after surgery.

course. The child took mesalamine (an anti-inflammatory) for a few years but stopped using it because he had no symptoms. He remained symptom-free until the past six months, when his family began to notice some bloating after meals. Lately, the bloating has become more uncomfortable, and occasionally the boy vomits after a meal. A few weeks ago, the child suffered from severe pain and vomiting after a meal and was checked by his GI doctor. A very narrowed part (stricture) of the ileum was seen on a special x-ray called a barium upper GI study (see chapter 8). The area of intestine before this narrowed part was dilated (enlarged), meaning the intestine above it had begun to stretch out as a result of the narrowing downstream. A colonoscopy (see chapter 9) was done, and this test showed a normal-looking colon. Medical therapy was recommended, and the barium x-ray was repeated, but there was no real change in the appearance of the narrowed area, and the symptoms stayed the same.

Why Surgery Might Be Right for This Child

There are a few reasons to believe that treatment with more medication will not work for this child. The fact that the intestine is dilated above the narrowing means that the stricture has been developing over a long time. The lack of change in the appearance of the intestine, even while he was on steroid therapy, shows that the narrowing may have become fixed like a scar (rather than just being due to inflamed tissue). In these circumstances, surgical treatment called *strictureplasty* might be a good option.

Strictureplasty widens the narrowed intestine to allow easier passage of intestinal contents, although it makes the intestines slightly shorter. The advantage of this type of operation is that the narrowing can be treated without removing a portion of the intestine. In addition, recovery might be faster than it would be if part of the intestine were removed.

Problems with this type of operation include the possibility of the stricture returning, and the possibility of fistula formation at the surgical site.

Scenario 3

A 10-year-old child has had recurrent abscesses (infections) around the anus for years. She was diagnosed with Crohn's disease and noted to have a stricture in the rectum, very close to the anus. Despite treatment with antibiotics, an immunomodulator medication, and then an anti-TNFα medication, the abscesses have continued and progressed. The stricture has gotten worse despite dilation by surgeons several times. When the abscesses are present, the child is in significant pain and is unable to sit up or lie on her back.

Why Surgery Might Be Right for This Child

In this case, the child has an aggressive *perianal* (around the anus) Crohn's disease. Perianal CD can be difficult to control with currently available medical treatments. Furthermore, taking out the involved parts of the intestine is a poor choice because the diseased areas are so low in the intestines that there is no bowel left to sew the good intestine to after removing the diseased part.

The complications of the perianal disease have severely affected this child's quality of life. As a result, an *intestinal diversion with ostomy* may be a good option for her. A diversion surgery involves cutting the intestine above where the severe disease is and bringing that part of intestine out through an opening in the skin (a stoma). Studies and experience have shown that moving the contents of the intestines away from diseased areas allows those areas to heal.

An enterostomal therapist assesses and counsels patients scheduled for diversion surgery. The nurse will tell the child and her family what to expect from the surgery, will fit the child with the appliance, and will help prepare everyone for life with the appliance. After the perianal disease is healed, doctors may decide to perform a *reanastomosis* (hook the intestine back together). The risk of recurrence after reanastomosis remains high, however, and the right choice might be to make the stoma permanent.

🔲 12

Managing Specific Problems

This chapter describes symptoms of an IBD flare, such as abdominal pain and rectal bleeding, as well as other health problems that a child with IBD might have. We discuss other causes (besides IBD) for each problem as appropriate, and we indicate what action parents might take when these problems occur. Many of the symptoms are also discussed in chapter 4.

Once a child receives a diagnosis of IBD, any new or repeated symptom naturally causes concern that the disease might be "acting up," or flaring. Intestinal symptoms need to be evaluated calmly, to find out whether they are related to IBD or other causes. A child with IBD can get abdominal symptoms (stomachache) for all the same reasons any child might, such as infections, gas, constipation, or indigestion. If one of your child's friends at school or a family member at home just had a stomach bug, that may be all that is going on.

Abdominal Pain

Abdominal pain is a very common complaint. Once your child reaches an age when she can describe her symptoms, it is always helpful to ask her to describe the pain in her own words. Sometimes the first question to ask is whether your child has felt this type of pain before. Even if she cannot describe it, she can usually answer this question. Children can often distinguish their IBD pain from other types of pain. If she cannot give you a word for the pain, ask about different sensations such as "pressure," "sharp," or "burning." Is the pain there all the time, or does it come and go? Did the pain start suddenly, or come on slowly? If the pain comes and goes, how long does it last each time?

Your child's doctor needs to know where the pain is and how intense it is. He also needs to know if the pain is always in the same place. Crohn's disease often involves the lower right side of the intestine, near where the appendix is located. Pain from the stomach is more likely to be felt above the navel (belly button), and pain from the colon is most likely to be felt nearer the middle of the abdomen.

The severity of pain, of course, depends on the person—some people seem to have high tolerance for pain; others are less tolerant. It is helpful to ask your child to compare this pain with past experience. You can also gauge the impact of your child's pain by how much it affects her activity, appetite, or sleep.

Try to determine if the pain is connected with anything. Does it only occur just before a bowel movement? Is it more likely to occur after eating, or with an empty stomach? Does anything help ease the pain, such as passing gas or stool? Does anything seem to make the pain worse? Pay particular attention if it seems that coughing or sneezing makes the pain worse. Does the abdomen seem unusually sensitive if you touch or rub it?

Your child may have significant symptoms, such as diarrhea, fever, or vomiting, that the doctor will need to hear about in detail. You should also mention more subtle or seemingly unrelated problems, such as mouth sores, joint pain, fatigue, or weight loss.

Carefully answering these questions with your child will help you and your child's doctor assess how severe and urgent the problem is, and whether immediate medical attention is needed:

- What does the pain feel like (pressure, sharp, burning, etc.)?
- Is the pain constant or does it come and go? For intermittent pain, how long does it last?
- Did the pain start suddenly or slowly?
- Where is the pain located?
- How much does it hurt compared to other abdominal pain in the past?

- Does the pain affect activities of daily living or sleep?
- Does anything make it better or worse?
- Does the pain get worse when the child coughs or sneezes?
- Is the abdomen sensitive to touch?
- Does the child have any other symptoms?

Call your child's doctor if severe, constant pain persists. Call your child's doctor if your child shows signs of unusual sensitivity to touch or motion. Watch to see if milder symptoms go away or continue, especially if they seem different from previous flares of IBD. When in doubt about abdominal pain, it is always best to call your child's doctor. The nurse or doctor can then help you decide if your child should be seen right away or if any tests should be done.

Rectal Bleeding

Blood in the stool is a common sign that IBD may be flaring. This symptom is never normal, but it is also not usually a reason to panic. Note how much blood is present, how often your child is having a bowel movement, and whether your child has diarrhea. Bloody diarrhea typically means that the colon is inflamed, and this inflammation can be due to an IBD flare. It is best to contact the doctor early on to rule out infection and decide about further testing and treatment. Rarely, a child may have significant bleeding. *If it seems that there is more blood than stool, seek medical attention immediately.*

If the blood is associated with no change in bowel habits, it may not be due to IBD. Patients in remission may become constipated, and passing hard stool can sometimes cause bleeding from a fissure (small tear or cut in the skin near the anus). People with CD can also develop inflammation around the anus as part of the disease, and their inflammation can cause bleeding.

Anemia

Persistent loss of blood in the stools (even in tiny or invisible amounts) can lead to low levels of hemoglobin, a condition called *anemia*. Hemoglobin is the part of the red blood cells that carries oxygen to the rest of the body. Anemia can be caused by direct loss of blood as well as by indirect loss of iron, which is an important part of hemoglobin.

IBD can cause anemia for other reasons in addition to blood loss. CD of the small intestine may cause iron to be poorly absorbed (taken into the body). The body needs iron to produce new blood cells, and therefore low iron levels can lead to anemia. Other vitamins are also important for the production of blood cells, and poor nutrition or poor absorption of these nutrients (for example, folic acid or vitamin B12) can also lead to anemia.

Mild anemia may not cause any symptoms. As blood counts fall below normal, however, the first symptom you will notice in your child is fatigue (tiredness). More severe anemia can cause dizziness or lightheadedness, shortness of breath, and rapid heart rate. Symptoms will come on more quickly, and be more intense, the faster the blood count falls. During routine visits, as well as during a flare of the disease, the doctor will check your child's blood counts. If your child's doctor recommends iron for treatment of the anemia, this can be done using oral or IV formulations.

Diarrhea

Diarrhea is another common, and often prominent, symptom of IBD, but not every loose stool is cause for concern. Everyone's bowel patterns can change naturally, especially with changes in diet. As with the stomach symptoms discussed earlier in this chapter, take the time to assess exactly what is happening with your child. Until your child has had a few episodes of diarrhea, he may not be able tell how abnormal his stool really is. You may need to insist on seeing it, even if he feels embarrassed by this request.

Make a note of how often the diarrhea occurs, whether it is associated with pain or cramps, and how loose it seems to be. The presence of blood with diarrhea is always an important sign. School-age children typically try not to have bowel movements in school, so if your child begins to have bowel movements at school, that may be a sign of diarrhea. Getting up at night for a bowel movement is a sign of more significant diarrhea. If there is significant diarrhea, bring a stool sample to the doctor's office or clinic.

The sample can be checked for hidden blood, then sent to the lab and checked for infection.

Systemic Symptoms

The signs and symptoms of IBD are not always confined to the digestive (gastrointestinal, or GI) tract. Symptoms of IBD may involve the body as a whole, in which case they are called *systemic symptoms*. Systemic symptoms may include fatigue, loss of appetite with associated weight loss, and fever. Children and adolescents may have slowed growth and delayed puberty.

These problems are largely the result of intestinal inflammation and the related problem of not getting enough calories from food. The immune system releases substances called *cytokines* during inflammation responses. Cytokines cause many systemic signs and symptoms even when the inflammation itself is so mild that there are no obvious GI symptoms.

Fatigue and Loss of Appetite

An important part of maintaining health in a child or adolescent with IBD is identifying and treating specific conditions that can contribute to fatigue, such as anemia or not eating enough calories. Certain cytokines can reduce appetite, and therefore a person having an inflammation response may not consume enough calories in her diet. Inflammation in the stomach (*gastritis*) can cause discomfort while eating, which again reduces appetite and the amount of food a person eats. Regardless of the cause, if a child is not getting enough calories, the result will be fatigue and weight loss (or poor weight gain), which lead to further harmful effects on her health. If she drinks liquid nutritional supplements during a time of active disease, she will have an easier time maintaining or gaining weight. Controlling the acid in the child's stomach with medications can ease some of the discomfort of eating.

Symptoms such as fatigue and loss of appetite can also be signs of the emotional, psychological (mental), and social effects of this disease, both before and after diagnosis. Fatigue and loss of appetite are common feelings that take a toll on quality of life in anyone with a chronic illness.

Fever

Fevers can be the result of another illness your child has while also having IBD. This other illness may require specific treatment in addition to the IBD treatment your child is receiving. Fevers associated with IBD are usually low grade and irregular. You can treat them with acetaminophen. Treatment with nonsteroidal anti-inflammatory drugs (NSAIDs), such as ibuprofen, is controversial and should be avoided when possible for fever. Ibuprofen can sometimes worsen IBD and should be taken only on a doctor's advice. These medications can cause additional injury to the digestive tract and may induce an IBD flare.

Delayed Puberty

Disease-related factors can affect growth and puberty (see chapter 4). Some of the most effective medications for treating inflammation—for example, steroids such as prednisone—can slow growth as well. Doctors try very hard to reduce the use of long-term steroids taken by mouth. Treating delayed growth and sexual development involves

- supporting good nutrition,
- treating the inflammation to reduce the release of cytokines, and
- minimizing the use of steroids.

Extraintestinal Manifestations

As discussed in earlier chapters, inflammatory bowel disease affects different portions of the digestive tract. Ulcerative colitis is limited to the large intestine, and Crohn's disease can affect any area between the mouth and the anus. It is not unusual for other parts of the body to be affected by IBD as well. When the disease involves areas beyond the digestive tract, the problems created by the IBD are called *extraintestinal manifestations* of inflammatory bowel disease. Some of these extraintestinal symptoms occur only when digestive tract inflammation is active, while others occur when there are no digestive tract symptoms. In the following sections, we discuss some of the extraintestinal manifestations of IBD.

Joints and Bones

Many children have joint pain (*arthralgia*) and arm and leg (*extremity*) pain, whether or not they have IBD. "Growing pains" are a common part of normal childhood, as are other causes of joint and bone pain, such as sports injuries. Nonetheless, extremity and joint pain can be specifically related to IBD or to the medications used to treat IBD. Joint pain can occur when the doctor decreases prednisone doses, or when a child starts taking immunosuppressant medications, such as azathioprine or 6-mercaptopurine. Joint pain associated with medication changes usually goes away over time and does not require treatment.

Joint inflammation (*arthritis*) occurs in up to 20 percent of adults with IBD, but it seems to affect children and teens less commonly. In contrast to joint pain, arthritis causes not only pain but also joint swelling and redness, and the joint might feel warm to the touch. Despite these symptoms, the types of arthritis associated with IBD rarely damage the affected joints. Nevertheless, you should *notify your child's IBD specialist immediately if a joint becomes red and swollen*, because it is important to rule out an infection in the joint. Depending on the type and severity of the arthritis, the doctor may want your child to be seen by a pediatric rheumatologist, an expert in children with arthritis.

Some types of IBD-related arthritis worsen only when the digestive tract symptoms worsen. In those cases, treating the digestive tract symptoms also effectively treats the arthritis. Pain medications with or without physical therapy may be prescribed while the digestive tract symptoms are treated. When arthritis occurs without digestive tract symptoms, treatment may involve physical therapy, pain medication, and medicines such as steroids, methotrexate, or infliximab to suppress the inflammation.

Ibuprofen and similar medicines to treat pain can worsen IBD, but some doctors will suggest trying these medications and continuing them if digestive tract symptoms do not worsen. You should discuss the risks and benefits of using ibuprofen and related pain-relief medications with your child's physician.

Rarely, the joints of the back can be affected by IBD in conditions called *sacroiliitis* and *ankylosing spondylitis*. Symptoms of these disorders include morning back stiffness, gradual low-back pain that is worse with rest, and pain spreading to the buttocks. These problems can occur even when there are no digestive tract symptoms. Should these symptoms develop, your child's IBD specialist may order x-rays and blood tests. Treatment of ankylosing spondylitis and sacroiliitis may include pain medications and immunosuppressant medications, such as methotrexate and infliximab. Your child's doctor will probably want your child to be examined by a pediatric rheumatologist.

Decreased bone density, called *osteopenia*, and a more severe condition, *osteoporosis*, are common in adults with IBD and can occur in children and adolescents with IBD as well. Considerably decreased bone density can increase the risk of broken bones (fractures). It is likely that many different factors affect bone density in IBD. Although more research is needed, factors thought to decrease bone density include

- steroid use
- insufficient calcium and vitamin D in the diet
- problems with absorption of calcium and vitamin D (the child gets enough calcium and vitamin D in the diet, but the body can't take it in and use it because the intestinal lining is damaged)
- inactivity
- alcohol use
- smoking
- digestive tract inflammation

The best way to prevent osteoporosis in children with IBD is still unknown. Getting enough calcium and vitamin D in the diet, avoiding alcohol and tobacco, and doing weight-bearing exercises regularly are all recommended. If your child has severe or persistent bone or back pain, you should notify the IBD specialist. An x-ray or other tests may be needed.

Some doctors recommend tests to screen for osteoporosis as part of routine care, while others do so only in specific situations.

Mouth and Skin

Mouth sores or mouth ulcers are common in children and adolescents with IBD, and many healthy children have them, too. In children with IBD, they tend to worsen during flares of digestive tract symptoms and improve when the digestive tract symptoms are treated. They may also go away without any particular treatment. Although the condition is generally more of an annoyance than a serious complication, mouth pain from the ulcers may cause children to eat poorly. Topical numbing mouthwashes can help decrease the discomfort associated with mouth sores and may make eating easier. Your child's doctor may recommend other medications or mouthwashes, if the topical numbing washes are not enough.

Rashes such as eczema, dry skin, and acne are common in children with and without IBD. Steroids may make acne worse in adolescents. In addition to these normal childhood rashes, children with IBD are at risk for other skin problems, such as *Erythema nodosum* and pyoderma gangrenosum. Both are relatively uncommon, particularly in children.

Erythema nodosum typically appears as red, painful bumps on the front of the lower legs. It tends to occur when digestive tract symptoms flare, and it goes away either on its own or as the digestive tract symptoms are treated.

Pyoderma gangrenosum begins as pustules (pus-filled bumps), often on the feet or lower legs. The pustules then develop into skin ulcerations. Ulcerations are usually painful, and they can be brought on or worsened by injury to the skin. They can occur without any digestive tract symptoms. Although they may go away on their own over several months, they are often treated with immunosuppressant medications such as steroids, cyclosporine (or related medications), or infliximab.

As explained elsewhere in this book, Crohn's disease often results in fissures, ulcers, and tags (thickened flaps of skin), mostly on the skin around the anus. Occasionally, similar problems occur on the skin of other areas of the body. This condition is referred to as *metastatic cutaneous*

Crohn's disease. Metastatic cutaneous CD can occur even when digestive tract symptoms are absent. Treatment of this condition often involves taking one or more immunosuppressant medications.

Eyes

We discuss eye problems in chapter 4. They are often treated with eye drops, but oral steroids or immunosuppressant medications may occasionally be needed. Steroids can cause other eye problems, such as glaucoma or cataracts, when used for long periods.

Liver Disease

This discussion provides information on the treatment of the liver conditions mentioned in chapter 4. A doctor may suspect liver disease when a child's liver function tests are abnormal. Liver function tests are blood tests that measure levels of certain liver enzymes, such as GGT, ALT, and AST. Another liver function test measures the level of bilirubin, a product of the breakdown of red blood cells (red blood cells are broken down in the liver).

To treat primary sclerosing cholangitis (PSC; inflammation of the bile ducts), doctors may prescribe ursodeoxycholate (ursodiol). Other anti-inflammatory and immunosuppressive treatments are sometimes used, but none has been conclusively proved to work. Some patients with severe PSC may need a liver transplant.

Gallstones often do not cause symptoms, and if any are found during an ultrasound, they do not need to be treated. Rarely, they might get stuck and cause symptoms in a bile duct, and then they need to be removed through an ERCP scope (see chapter 9). If inflammation of the gallbladder develops (if the child has a "gallbladder attack"), the gallbladder (often with gallstones inside) will need to be surgically removed. This can be done safely through a laparoscopy in almost all patients, even after surgery for CD. A laparoscopy is surgery through the belly button; it involves smaller incisions (cuts) and quicker recovery than laparotomy. Because the gallbladder stores, concentrates, and releases bile, removing bile after surgery may require more frequent, smaller meals that are low in fat to avoid diarrhea.

Nonalcoholic fatty liver disease (NAFLD) can occur with extended use of steroids, severe or sudden weight gain or weight loss, or too much *total parenteral nutrition* (TPN), a form of intravenous nutrition. The liver may become enlarged, with abnormal collections of fat inside the liver cells. NAFLD usually clears if a person

- follows a healthy diet
- takes ursodiol and vitamin E
- decreases steroid use
- reaches and maintains a normal weight

If NAFLD is severe or long-standing, however, cirrhosis and its complications can occur, though this is rare. Cirrhosis is scarring of the liver, which causes permanent liver damage.

Medications used to treat IBD, including azathioprine and 6-MP, can cause *drug-related hepatitis* (inflammation of the liver) in some children, due to individual differences in how the body processes these drugs. If your child develops hepatitis while taking any of these medicines, the doctor may decrease the dose or stop that particular medicine altogether. People taking these drugs should have their medication levels and liver functions regularly monitored by their physician. This is done through blood tests.

Kidney Problems

IBD is associated with a greater than average risk of developing certain kidney diseases. People with CD, especially those whose bodies malabsorb fat, may develop kidney stones. (Fat malabsorption occurs when the body cannot take in the fat that a person eats.) These stones may cause no symptoms, but sometimes they cause severe pain, blood in the urine, and decreased urination due to obstruction. Kidney stones may also damage the kidneys. Maintaining good control of CD, eating a healthy low-fat diet, and drinking lots of water (to avoid dehydration) helps prevent kidney stones. If they develop, there are different approaches to treating them. Stones sometimes pass out of the body on their own (in the urine), but if they do not, then medications can be taken or the stones can be removed by inserting an endoscope through an incision (in *keyhole surgery*) or using *lithotripsy*. Lithotripsy is a noninvasive procedure done while the patient is sedated or under anesthesia. A focused high-intensity acoustic pulse is applied through the skin in an attempt to break up the stones, to make them small enough to pass out of the body through the ureters.

Cyclosporine and tacrolimus are medications that a doctor might prescribe to treat severe UC and, rarely, severe CD. These medicines can directly damage the kidneys, especially at higher doses or if they are used for a long time. If your child is taking these medications, he must take them *exactly* as they have been prescribed and must have regular blood tests to check the level of the medication in the blood and to check kidney function. Careful monitoring is needed to avoid permanent kidney damage, high blood pressure, and kidney failure. A person with kidney failure requires dialysis or a kidney transplant.

Some people with IBD have an increased risk of developing a form of kidney inflammation called *tubular interstitial nephritis*, which can cause the kidneys to stop working. Medications containing 5-aminosalicylates (5-ASA), such as mesalamine, olsalazine, balsalazide, and sulfasalazine, can increase the risk of developing this problem. Although most doctors do not routinely check blood levels of these medications, if your child is taking these drugs, he should have regular urinalysis and blood tests to check creatinine levels (a kidney function test). If abnormalities are found, he should stop taking the medicines in order to prevent permanent kidney damage.

Rarely, during a difficult pelvic surgery for UC, such as a pouch procedure, the ureters (the tubes connecting the kidney to the bladder) are damaged. If this happens, the ureters will require surgical repair. During this surgery, there may also be damage to the nerves of the bladder or the urogenital system. This nerve damage can lead to urinary incontinence or impotence (in males). This surgical complication is rare, but it is a recognized risk and is not always correctable if it occurs.

Bladder Problems

CD can affect the bladder. When children experience the symptoms of urinary tract infection—pain or a burning sensation during urination—

the cause of these symptoms may be irritation from an adjacent inflamed part of the bowel or a fistula connecting the intestine to the bladder. When a child has irritation, a urine test may reveal an increase in white blood cells (the cells that are involved in the inflammatory process and in fighting infections). In irritation, no bacteria are found in a urine test. When a child has a fistula, a urine test may reveal air, blood, and even small remains of stool as well as bacteria.

In children with CD, a fistula (abnormal opening) sometimes develops between the digestive tract and the bladder, which can lead to infection. Radiographic studies such as abdominal CT scan or magnetic resonance imaging (MRI) may identify the fistula. Surgery might be necessary to treat this complication of the disease.

In many children with a fistula to the bladder, urinary tract infections tend to come back, but serious complications, such as kidney infections, are very rare. A fistula can be identified on a barium x-ray, a CT scan, or direct examination of the bladder by a physician looking through a *cystoscope* (a device similar to the endoscope but with a very slim tube).

Antibiotics and anti-inflammatory medicines (such as steroids or azathioprine) may be effective in treating bladder problems. When a fistula is present, or when symptoms do not go away with medical therapy, surgical removal of the inflamed part of the bowel, and the fistula, will solve the problem. Special diets are not very helpful in the treatment of these problems.

Strictures

Strictures, or narrowing of the bowel due to inflammation and scarring, are very common in CD. If they cause no symptoms, they might be discovered only during a barium test (see chapter 8). Strictures can cause symptoms, however, including cramping pain, bloating, nausea, vomiting, and less frequent, less satisfactory bowel movements. These symptoms result when the flow of intestinal contents is blocked. If these symptoms occur, let your child's doctor know immediately. Rarely, infection and reduced blood flow to the bowel can result from strictures, and these problems require medication or surgery.

For an acute obstruction, usually a short period of bowel "rest" (no food or drink by mouth), intravenous fluids, and steroids relieve stricture-related obstruction without the need for surgery to remove the affected area, although surgery may sometimes be necessary. If the narrowed area is within the reach of an endoscope, the doctor may place a stent or inject steroids directly into the stricture to try to prevent a return of the problem. If the stricture is long, surgery to widen the opening through the intestine (called strictureplasty) can be done, often laparoscopically (through the belly button). Doctors recommend this surgery to relieve the symptoms of chronic or recurrent obstruction, while avoiding the possible loss of too much bowel. (Losing too much bowel can lead to a problem known as *short bowel syndrome.*)

If your child has an intestinal stricture, the following tips can help her reduce the risk of obstruction:

- Avoid high-roughage foods like nuts and popcorn.
- Chew food completely.
- Drink plenty of fluids with meals.
- Eat smaller meals more frequently.
- Avoid capsule endoscopy (pill camera; see chapter 8), because the camera capsule can get stuck.

Abscess

An abscess, or local infection, is rare in children with UC and more common in children with CD. Symptoms vary by the site of the abscess. They include fever, chills, lethargy, and pain. Other symptoms are tenderness, redness, and warmth in the area or in the skin above it, as well as drainage (oozing). If these symptoms occur, tell your child's doctor immediately because sepsis, a severe bodywide infection in the bloodstream, may occur. A CT scan or MRI scan (see chapter 8) might help diagnose an abscess if it is in the abdomen or pelvis, and blood tests often show an elevated white blood cell count. (An elevated WBC indicates an infection.)

Children who have recently had surgery or other procedures, and those who have a fistula, are at higher risk of getting an abscess. Another risk factor is taking medications that suppress the immune system, especially at high doses or for long periods. Children with suppressed immune systems may have more subtle signs of an abscess at first, but they may get sicker from it.

If your child has an abscess, the doctor may put him on antibiotics by mouth or by IV (through the vein). In some cases, a surgeon may have to drain the abscess. A radiologist with a needle guided by ultrasound or CT scan can also drain an abscess. When an abscess affects the skin, wound care experts may provide additional advice. Keeping the area clean, dry, and protected often helps with healing.

Fistula

Fistula, an abnormal opening or connection between the digestive tract and other organs, typically occurs in CD. Only very rarely do fistulas develop in children with UC, most often after pouch surgery. If a fistula happens after pouch surgery, pouch correction and removal are frequently required (resulting in the need for permanent ileostomy; see chapter 11).

A fistula can also result from or lead to infection, including the development of an abscess. Symptoms of fistula vary greatly, as do the treatment options and their success rates. Symptoms and treatments of fistulas depend on their location, number, and size, as well as on how long the fistula was present before treatment and whether it is internal (inside the body) or external (opens onto the skin).

In CD, fistulas from the intestine to the skin and tissues around the anus are common and are easier to treat than other fistulas. Symptoms include pain, irritation, and swelling. Drainage of stool, blood, and pus can occur, making sitting and walking uncomfortable.

Pain control is an important part of treating fistulas. There are many new and improved treatments available. Antibiotics (ciprofloxacin and metronidazole) are effective in decreasing symptoms and healing fistulas, but when these treatments stop, recurrence is common. Once any infection is cleared, antibiotic therapy might be followed by infliximab, or by cyclosporine or tacrolimus. The surgeon may place a *seton* (a piece of fabric, thread, or a small plastic wick) in the fistulous tract to promote healing, particularly in patients with an abscess. Fibrin "glue" can also help close the opening.

It is not always possible to achieve lasting healing of the fistula, even with infliximab, the most effective therapy. Incomplete closure may be acceptable if a child is otherwise doing well. Once the fistula is closed, continuous treatment with infliximab, 6-MP, or azathioprine will likely be required to prevent recurrence.

Diagnosis of other types of fistulas can be difficult and requires a combination of tests, including barium x-rays, CT scan, MRI, ultrasound, and endoscopy or colonoscopy. These tests may require anesthesia to avoid discomfort. Very rarely, a fistula develops that connects the rectum and the vagina, or other organs of the reproductive tract, such as the fallopian tubes and ovaries. These types of fistulas are particularly difficult to treat and potentially very harmful socially. They can also cause severe problems when a woman tries to become pregnant. A stoma (see chapter 11) or many surgeries, combined with medications, are often necessary to treat fistulas involving the reproductive organs.

Internal fistulas from one diseased bowel area to another may not cause any symptoms and may not require treatment. Surgery to remove the connected segments might be needed, however, if symptoms occur or if the fistula connects to the bladder or the urinary tract, causing repeated infections.

Perforation

A perforation of the intestine occurs when the wall of the intestine develops a hole, allowing the contents of the intestine (especially bacteria) to spill into nearby spaces and organs. A perforation may result in the formation of an abscess or in a more general infection of the abdominal cavity (called *peritonitis*). A perforation causing a localized abscess is called a *walled-off perforation*. This happens when a nearby structure (such as the intestine itself, the bladder, or the uterus) seals off the perforation. A perforation resulting in peritonitis is called a *free perforation*.

Free perforations are uncommon in IBD. In CD, perforations usually occur in the small bowel, are generally walled off, and may be the first symptom of the disease. In UC, free perforations can occur in the large bowel (colon) and are likely to cause peritonitis.

The main risk factors leading to perforations are severe inflammation and enlarged segments of bowel that are ahead of a stricture. Your child's doctor will suspect a perforation if your child suddenly develops abdominal tenderness, pain, and fever. A new mass (lump), detected during a physical exam, can also be a sign of perforation.

When the doctor suspects a perforation, she will order tests such as abdominal x-ray, ultrasound, CT scan, or MRI of the abdomen to examine the intestine and the abdominal area. If the doctor finds a perforation, treatment will usually begin with antibiotics to control any possible infection. When there is a free perforation, immediate surgery may be required to seal it off. In these cases, it is likely that no food by mouth will be allowed until your child recovers from the surgery, and feeding will be done through a vein.

When a child has a walled-off perforation, surgery may be required to either drain the abscess or remove the diseased portion of intestine. The timing of the surgery will depend on the response to treatment. If your child is having severe pain with a regular diet, switching to a liquid formula may help.

IBD experts believe that perforation is a feature of a CD subgroup. Patients with this type of Crohn's disease are at higher risk of repeated fistulas or perforation. At present, there is no known way to prevent this complication.

Cancer

One of the long-term complications of IBD is colon cancer, which is tied to the chronic inflammation of the colon whether the diagnosis is UC or CD. The risk of developing colon cancer depends on several factors, including how long the person has had IBD and how severe the inflammation of the colon is. The risk increases beyond the risk of the general population once a person has had the disease for more than eight or ten years. The cancer risk does not go away even if the disease remains inactive (in remission), but there is some growing evidence that keeping the disease in remission can actually help decrease the cancer risk.

Taking this risk into account, once the disease has been present for approximately eight to ten years, regular screening for colon cancer must begin. Most children with IBD are diagnosed in their teens, so this concern does not often come up until the college years or early adulthood. Monitoring includes annual checkups with a gastroenterologist and regular colonoscopies with biopsies to look for the early signs of cancer.

Researchers are constantly looking for new, less invasive ways to detect cancer early. It is likely that in the not-too-distant future, we will monitor for cancer by testing blood or stool, instead of with a colonoscopy. CT scans and MRI imaging are already nearly as effective as a colonoscopy at detecting polyps and colon cancer. As new testing becomes available, the screening recommendations will change.

▣ 13

The Role of Nutrition

Just as a builder must have tools to make a house, children's bodies must have food to help them grow and to give them energy to play and do schoolwork. When children are sick, food becomes even more important, because good nutrition is necessary to help them get better.

Doctors and dieticians often use the word *nutrition* when they talk about the benefits of food. Nutrition includes proteins, carbohydrates, fats, and other important materials such as vitamins and minerals. When your child has inflammatory bowel disease, she needs good nutrition to get better. Your child's doctor will recommend many helpful and healthy foods for your child. If your child cannot eat all the recommended foods, the doctor will suggest some nutritional supplements.

The first symptoms of IBD in children and adolescents often include weight loss or failure to gain weight at a normal rate. Many people who have IBD find it difficult to eat enough good food. They may feel hungry, but when it is time to eat, they can finish only a small amount. Food may not taste good, or they may just find it difficult to eat. Some people get stomachaches or diarrhea after eating, so they stop eating in order to avoid these symptoms.

An inflamed, swollen portion of the intestine acts as a funnel through which food and gas must pass. As they pass, the thickened (and sometimes ulcerated) bowel stretches, causing pain or other unpleasant symptoms. By eating less, children decrease the food-related symptoms. For those with Crohn's disease, a severe narrowing of the gut can cause even worse symptoms.

If a child does not eat well for a long time, weight loss, slow growth, and delayed puberty can result. In addition, intestinal inflammation symptoms can become worse when a person does not eat, because the body lacks the building blocks necessary to heal the intestine.

Nutrition is important to a child's whole body, including the digestive tract—the mouth, stomach, and small and large intestines. Therefore, most doctors try to supply the gastrointestinal (GI) tract with nutrients. In the past, doctors thought that not putting any food in the GI tract would help it heal by giving it a rest, and they would prescribe nothing to eat (but plenty of fluids) for several weeks. They found, however, that the digestive tract needs food just as much as the rest of the body. Doctors no longer prescribe "bowel rest" except in rare situations.

Because of the eating and nutritional problems of people with IBD, the doctor may pay special attention to your child's bones. Normally, bones become stronger as a child grows and continue to get stronger until a person reaches his midtwenties. Several factors, however, can cause children with IBD to have weaker bones than normal:

- Children with IBD may not get enough minerals, such as calcium and phosphorus, or vitamins, such as vitamin D. This occurs for two reasons: they are not consuming adequate amounts, and they may have some degree of malabsorption. These minerals and vitamins are necessary for strong, healthy bones.
- Some medications, such as steroids, can weaken bones. Your child may need to take extra vitamins and minerals.

The doctor may request a special test for your child, to check bone strength. The test is called DEXA (dual-energy x-ray absorptiometry).

Caloric Requirements

According to some reports, children with IBD symptoms sometimes eat only about half the calories they require for their age. Yet, children and teens with IBD need 20 to 40 percent more energy than children who do not have IBD. This figure is based on the estimated energy requirements

(EER) for healthy children. The EER is the amount of energy that the Food and Nutrition Board considers sufficient to meet the known needs of most healthy people. This amount will vary depending on a child's size, age, and stage of development.

As a rough estimate, children with IBD need about 2,000 to 2,200 calories every day for girls, and 2,300 to 2,600 calories every day for boys. Your doctor will tell you what your child's caloric needs are, or your doctor may ask a dietician to help you figure out how many calories your child needs. The dietician can show you what foods will help give your child the necessary calories.

Protein and calories work together. Because your child needs the right combination of both, his doctor or dietician will also recommend how much protein he should be consuming daily. Medications that undo the inflammation increase the width of the gut, allowing food to pass more easily. When treatment starts, some children find it easier to eat several small meals and snacks in a day, rather than three regular meals. Making sure that a child gets enough calories and protein to continue growing is more important than the number of meals she eats. The recommended goals for weight gain will depend on the child's age, sex, and degree of undernutrition.

Specific Nutrients

Iron

Apart from overall inadequate caloric intake, the most common nutritional problem for children and teenagers with IBD is iron deficiency. Iron deficiency can lead to anemia (low red blood cell count). This deficiency occurs for several reasons in people with IBD, including not getting enough iron from food, decreased iron absorption in the gut, and increased iron losses from the intestine due to visible bleeding or hidden (occult) bleeding. Doctors usually diagnose iron-deficiency anemia using a routine blood test and treat the anemia with iron supplements.

Calcium

Calcium is an essential part of bones. Along with phosphorus, it gives bones their strength. Calcium also plays important roles in passing nerve signals along and in muscle contraction.

All people with IBD, and especially growing children, must consume their daily requirement of calcium. This will help ensure the normal development of their bones and prevent osteoporosis in the future. Calcium requirements change with age and are highest in children entering puberty, a time when they are growing fast. There are several guidelines for calcium requirements in children. In general, for children between ages 3 and 8 years, 500 to 800 mg of calcium per day is recommended, whereas children aged 9 to 18 years should get 1,200 to 1,300 mg each day.

Calcium occurs naturally in a variety of foods, and most people with IBD can absorb calcium normally from the intestine. The most important dietary source of calcium is dairy products. One cup of milk or yogurt contains 300 mg of calcium, and 1 ounce of natural or processed cheese has 200 mg of calcium. Other foods that contain calcium, although less of it, are

- canned fish with bones (250 mg in 3 oz)
- corn tortillas
- calcium-set tofu
- Chinese cabbage
- kale
- broccoli

Some people reduce their intake of dairy and calcium because of symptoms of lactose intolerance (inability to digest foods containing lactose). To avoid this problem, they can choose lactose-free products and dairy products that have low lactose content and still have a good level of calcium. These include aged cheeses, cottage cheese, kefir cultured milk drink, processed and natural cheeses, and yogurt with live cultures. Many juices are now fortified with calcium and offer an alternative to milk (they may contain 320 mg of calcium in each cup). Soda and other soft drinks do not contain calcium. Children who drink soda instead of milk may not get enough calcium in their diet.

Some medications used to treat IBD, especially corticosteroids, can affect the absorption of calcium, and when used long term, they can affect bone strength. Although corticosteroids are excellent medications to bring about remission in IBD, they do not work well to maintain remission. Therefore, after your child feels better, the doctor will use medications that offer the possibility of long-term remission without the unwelcome side effects of corticosteroids. This approach should help minimize the effect of corticosteroids on bone health as well. If your child cannot stop taking corticosteroids, taking them every other day will minimize their side effects while maintaining their benefits.

Lactose

Lactose is the sugar found in the milk of mammals. It is found in human and cow's milk and in any dairy product derived from milk. Lactose intolerance is a condition that causes abdominal pain, diarrhea, or gas after eating or drinking something with lactose in it. These symptoms occur when someone does not have enough *lactase*, the intestinal enzyme that digests (breaks down) lactose. An intestinal enzyme is a special type of protein located on the lining of the intestines.

Many people think they should avoid lactose if they have IBD. Studies have shown, however, that lactose intolerance is no more common among people with IBD than among people without IBD. Therefore, your child should not restrict dairy products unless he has proved lactose intolerance. Even then, studies show that most people with real lactose intolerance can drink about 8 ounces of milk (1 cup) without having symptoms.

If your child has lactose intolerance and drinks lactose, it will not harm his body. He may experience loose stools or some gas and abdominal discomfort, but these symptoms will stop after an hour or two. Tablets that contain lactase (the enzyme that breaks down milk sugar) can be taken to help minimize or eliminate the symptoms that might otherwise occur. Your child can take the tablets before eating or drinking foods that contain lactose, or he can drink milk that is treated with the enzyme lactase to remove lactose.

If you think your child has symptoms with lactose ingestion, ask his doctor about available tests to diagnose lactose intolerance. Sometimes it is difficult to eliminate all dairy products from a diet without the help of a dietician. There is no reason to deny your child desirable dairy food if he is not lactose intolerant.

Fiber

Fiber is made of plant materials that humans cannot digest. It helps regulate bowel movements and prevent diseases such as cancer, heart disease, obesity, and diabetes. Unfortunately, most Americans do not eat enough fiber. Unless your child's doctor thinks your child should not have fiber, there is no reason to limit fiber-containing foods just because your child has IBD. The National Academy of Sciences recommends that children between the ages of 9 and 18 have 29 to 38 grams of fiber every day.

Vitamin D

Vitamin D helps the body absorb calcium in the intestine and helps maintain a healthy immune system. The body produces vitamin D naturally when the skin is exposed to sunlight. The daily requirement of vitamin D is 400 IU (international units) each day or 800 IU each day when exposure to sunlight is limited. Few foods are a natural source of vitamin D; some foods are fortified (have added vitamin D).

Foods that naturally contain vitamin D include fish liver oils, flesh of fatty fish (such as salmon and herring), and eggs (from hens that have been fed vitamin D). In the United States, milk is fortified with vitamin D (400 IU/quart), and cereals are also fortified.

Vitamin D production in the skin is the body's major natural source of this important nutrient. Natural sunlight stimulates production of the vitamin in the skin. Children who do not feel well and stay indoors a lot are at risk for vitamin D deficiency. In addition, children living in northern areas have lower vitamin D levels in the fall and winter, due to lack of exposure to sunlight.

Skin protected by sunblock lotions or creams will produce only a little of the vitamin. Exposure to sunlight shining through glass windows is not enough to stimulate vitamin D production in the skin. Only sensible exposure of unprotected skin to natural sunlight can ensure an adequate supply of this vitamin. In general, however, using sunblock is recommended to protect against skin cancer.

Folic Acid

Folic acid is a form of vitamin B. Sources of folic acid include

- enriched cereal grains
- dark leafy vegetables
- enriched and whole-grain breads and bread products
- fortified ready-to-eat cereals

People who do not have enough folic acid (folic acid deficiency) may develop anemia (low number of red blood cells). People with IBD who take sulfasalazine (a medication that treats colon inflammation) can develop folic acid deficiency. Daily folic acid supplements, given in tablet form, can correct this deficiency. These tablets are available over the counter. Folic acid should also be given to anyone receiving methotrexate treatment.

Folic acid may play a role in reducing long-term colon cancer risk in people with IBD (particularly UC), although more studies are needed on this subject. Another possible benefit of folic acid supplements may be a decrease in homocysteine levels. Homocysteine is a chemical that has been linked to cardiovascular (heart) disease and to the risk of thrombosis (blood clots).

Vitamin B12

Vitamin B12 is found in fortified cereals, meat, fish, and poultry; it is specifically absorbed in the lower ileum (the last part of the small intestine). Patients with IBD who have an inflamed lower ileum (*ileitis*), or who have had surgery to remove this part of the intestine, are at risk for vitamin B12 deficiency. Prolonged vitamin B12 deficiency leads to anemia and nerve damage. This deficiency can take months or years to develop because the body stores a large amount of vitamin B12 in the liver, and it takes time to exhaust this supply. The doctor can measure the amount of vitamin B12 in your child's body with a blood test. This will determine if your child needs vitamin B12 supplements. A vitamin B12 gel given into the nose, or monthly injections of vitamin B12, can correct a deficiency if it develops.

Zinc

Zinc is another important element for the body. It is necessary to help your child grow normally, and for her body to heal. It may even protect against infections. Zinc is lost in diarrhea; the more diarrhea your child has, the more zinc she will lose. Your child's doctor may check blood for zinc levels and, depending on the result, recommend that she take a zinc supplement.

Other Vitamins and Minerals

Many specialists recommend that children with IBD take multivitamin and mineral supplements daily because of reports of certain deficiencies in children with this disease. For example, 1 out of 8 children with IBD has a deficiency in vitamin A and vitamin E. Oral vitamin supplements can correct or prevent these deficiencies in most people.

Some studies suggest that children with IBD may benefit from taking antioxidants such as vitamin E, although more studies are needed to confirm whether there is a real benefit to this supplement.

Vitamin K, an important factor in normal blood clotting, is also active in bone. Mild vitamin K deficiency may play a role in bone loss in IBD.

Children with IBD may also have mineral deficiencies, especially during disease exacerbations (worsening). For example, people with chronic diarrhea may lose potassium and magnesium in their stool. Someone with a shortened gut after surgical removal of the intestines is at risk for electrolyte imbalances. Electrolytes are minerals dissolved in bodily fluids. They can often be replaced by consuming specialized drinks, such as sports drinks, that contain sodium and potassium.

Special Nutritional Formula

We know that nutritional status, particularly not getting enough nutrition, complicates the course of inflammatory bowel disease and changes the effectiveness of treatments. If your child has trouble getting enough food by mouth and is unable to keep up normal bodily functions (including a normal growth and immune response), he needs to be fed through other means. Nutritional support can be beneficial for a child with either UC or CD, especially if the child is not growing enough, or is undernourished.

In ulcerative colitis, *enteral nutrition*, a term that typically means nutrition using liquid foods (formulas), is usually a supplement to the child's regular diet. Enteral nutrition helps the child either catch up on lost weight or keep himself well nourished through a period of serious illness. Enteral nutritional support can also be one form of treatment for children with Crohn's disease (chapter 10).

Enteral Nutrition Support

Enteral nutrition can be taken by mouth, but repeatedly drinking the same liquid foods (formulas) may become tedious or difficult for a child. In these situations, tube feedings are an alternative way to administer the formulas that have all the nutrition your child needs to get better. Best of all, tube feedings can be done overnight. Many people find it reassuring to receive all the nutrition they need while they sleep. They are then free during the day to join their friends and family at the table without worrying about eating more than they feel they can. The tube delivers the formula directly into the intestinal tract (including the stomach and the first part of the small intestine, just past the stomach; figure 13.1). Enteral nutrition is an important treatment option that is available to all people with IBD.

A tube that starts in the nose and goes into the stomach (known as a *nasogastric tube*, or *NG tube*) can deliver enteral nutrition support, as can a tube that starts in the nose and goes into the small intestine (called a *nasojejunal tube*, or *NJ tube*). A tube that is surgically placed directly into the stomach (*gastrostomy tube*, or *G tube*) or into the small intestine (*jeju-*

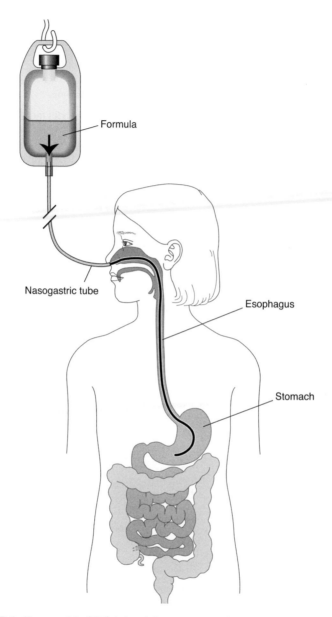

Figure 13.1. Nasogastric (NG) tube delivering enteral nutrition. People receiving enteral nutrition learn to pass a small flexible tube through their nasal cavity and esophagus and into the stomach. The tube can then be used to deliver supplemental formula. The formula is sometimes delivered at night by a small pump while the person is asleep.

Table 13.1
Types of tubes for enteral nutrition

Tube type	Abbreviation	Location
Nasogastric	NG tube	Starts in the nose and goes into the stomach
Nasojejunal	NJ tube	Starts in the nose and goes into the second part of the small intestine (jejunum)
Gastrostomy	G tube	Goes through the wall of the abdomen and into the stomach
Jejunostomy	J tube	Goes through the wall of the abdomen and into the jejunum

nostomy tube, or *J tube*) can also deliver this type of nutrition (table 13.1). Each route of entry into the gastrointestinal system has its advantages and disadvantages.

A tube placed through the nose is initially uncomfortable. Children resist the insertion of the tube, sometimes making it more difficult to thread it into the stomach. Once in place, the tube tends to cause some discomfort and irritation in the back of the nose and throat. Nonetheless, most children who decide to use this treatment adapt, and within a few minutes or hours, they accept the tube and move on to other activities. Often children will place NG tubes into their stomach at night before going to bed, thus using the tube and obtaining the extra nutrition while asleep. They remove the tube in the morning when they wake up. This way, they can go to school and participate in other activities without the tube in place.

An NJ tube, placed through the nose into the middle of the small intestine (jejunum), is more difficult to manage. Making sure the tube is in the proper position often involves an x-ray. The x-ray helps to make sure the tube is in the intestine and not in the stomach. Therefore, the NJ tube cannot be removed daily as an NG tube can. Despite good positioning within the intestine, NJ tubes may come back into the stomach. Children might even vomit out the tube, requiring that it be replaced using a similar process as described previously to ensure that the tube is in the proper position.

Doctors can insert tubes surgically through the skin and muscles of the abdominal wall, directly into the stomach or small intestine. That way, the tube does not have to pass down from the nose. Stomach tubes are usually placed by endoscopy in a short procedure called *percutaneous endoscopic gastrostomy* (PEG). The PEG procedure is relatively safe. Most of the time, a small tube that is almost flat to the skin of the abdomen can be used, although sometimes a longer tube is needed. The tubes are fairly easy to change when necessary, which may be every two to six months (or longer). Tubes are changed when they break, or when they become too tight and a larger size is needed.

Tubes that pass through the nose are kept in place with tape or other types of adhesives. If they slip out, the tube should be repositioned or completely replaced. Gastrostomy and jejunostomy tubes are held in place by a balloon or plastic dome within the stomach or intestine. The balloon can inadvertently deflate, which may cause the tube to come out. Should this happen, the tube should be replaced immediately so that the hole into the stomach or into the jejunum does not close. If the tube is difficult to replace or cannot be replaced, notify your child's doctor and take your child to the emergency room.

Once a tube is in place and provides access to the GI tract, it can be used for nourishment. Sometimes the tube is used only for giving medication or fluid (such as water). In most cases of IBD, however, the tube is used for formula feeding. The formula is given through the tube either all at once, like drinking a glass of milk, or, more typically, by a constant drip using a pump.

Many formulas are commercially available to use with feeding tubes. Formulas vary in composition, providing different amounts of calories and different types and proportions of carbohydrates, protein, and fat. Formulas also provide various amounts of other nutrients, including vitamins, trace elements (such as iron and zinc), and minerals (such as calcium).

The type of protein is often a major difference between formulas. Some formulas have protein that is whole, just like eating regular food or milk.

Other formulas have *predigested* protein. Predigested proteins are easier to digest and stimulate the immune system less. There are also formulas made of amino acids (the building blocks of proteins) and other nutrients that are easily absorbed, and these require minimal digestion. The formula may also contain other food substances, such as omega-3 fatty acids, glutamine, or fiber, that some doctors believe help patients who have IBD.

Complications of tubes are usually minor:

- The tape holding the tube in place can irritate the skin.
- Gastrostomy and jejunostomy tubes can leak acid or other intestinal fluids.
- Sometimes the tubes, especially the NG or NJ tubes, do not stay in a good position. This can lead to discomfort, nausea, vomiting, or chest or stomach pains.
- Diarrhea can occur, depending on the type of formula in use.

Less common problems include abnormal blood tests (electrolyte or other chemical imbalances) and aspiration—inhaling food into the lungs (possibly due to vomiting).

Parenteral Nutrition Support

Parenteral nutrition support is nutrition provided intravenously (through the vein). Enteral nutrition support costs less and has milder complications than parenteral nutrition, so enteral nutrition support is preferable to parenteral nutrition support. Occasionally, however, a child requires parenteral nutrition support.

Intravenous nutrition may be complete (total parenteral nutrition, or TPN) or supplemental. Supplemental parenteral nutrition is used in addition to enteral nutrition or to normal eating by mouth. Although parenteral nutrition usually starts in the hospital, many children are able to go home and lead normal lives (including participation in swimming and most other sports) while receiving parenteral nutrition support. Many home care companies are available throughout the world to assist children and their families with this treatment.

Parenteral nutrition is used for children whose intestinal system will not allow them to absorb or take in all the nutrients they need. Examples include

- children before or after surgery
- children who are severely malnourished
- children whose disease is complicated by
    fistula or fistulas
    short bowel syndrome
    toxic megacolon (a dangerously enlarged colon)
    intestinal obstruction (blockage) or perforation (hole)

Some children receive parenteral nutrition as part of treatment for Crohn's disease.

A catheter (tube) that leads into a vein provides parenteral nutrition. The vein may be a small vein (for example, in the arm), or it may be a large central vein (for example, the vena cava, near the heart; figure 13.2). Central veins must be used with long-term parenteral nutrition. This type of nutrition is often given at night by pump, while the child is asleep.

Parenteral nutrition requires a special sterile solution. The solution contains protein, fat, and glucose (sugar) as well as other nutrients, such as vitamins, minerals, and trace elements (table 13.2). These nutrients maintain health, including children's normal growth and development. Parenteral nutrition solutions can also include some medications (such as antacid medicines).

Complications of parenteral nutrition can be serious, so doctors select patients very carefully for this treatment. Before sending patients home, doctors must make sure that children, parents, and other caregivers receive proper training in the procedures involved with parenteral nutrition.

Complications of TPN can include

- an infection that enters the bloodstream (bactericidal or sepsis), which is the most serious complication
- blood clot (*thrombosis*) of the blood vessel where the catheter is located
- problems due to unusual fluid losses (such as severe diarrhea)
- glucose imbalances (high blood sugar or low blood sugar)

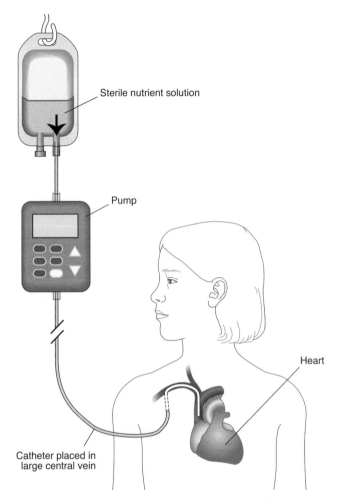

Figure 13.2. Catheter delivering parenteral nutrition. Rarely, children with IBD may be unable to eat, and they then require nutrition given by vein. Sterile nutrients in bags are delivered by pump into a large vein near the heart.

Monitoring Enteral and Parenteral Nutrition

Proper monitoring of enteral and parenteral nutrition support is essential to make sure that treatment is effective. Monitoring also ensures that the treatment is helping to achieve the goals set when the feedings started. In addition, monitoring prevents problems from occurring or getting worse.

Table 13.2
Composition of parenteral nutrition solutions

Nutrients

Water

Carbohydrate (glucose)

Fat (soybean/safflower oil)

Protein (simple amino acids)

Minerals: sodium, potassium, chloride, acetate, phosphorus, calcium, magnesium

Vitamins: for example, A, thiamine, riboflavin, niacin, pyridoxine, folate, cobalamin (B_{12}), pantothenate, biotin, C, D, E, K

Trace elements: zinc, copper, manganese, chromium, selenium

Medications (optional)

Antacid

Insulin

Heparin

Other medicines

Parents and other caregivers must watch the child for symptoms or signs of problems, to try to avoid complications. For example, any fever, persistent diarrhea, or vomiting should trigger a call to the doctor, and your child should be seen in the office or in the emergency room. Health care teams always monitor growth and disease activity in children with IBD, but they pay special attention to these factors when children receive special nutritional support.

Disease-Specific Nutrition Considerations

Ulcerative Colitis

Enteral or parenteral nutrition support by itself is typically not an effective treatment for a child with UC. Treatment in these children relies on medicine or surgery, while the nutritional treatment is usually a supplement for support. Often the nutrition support starts while a child is in the hospital for a serious flare of colitis. In addition to intravenous fluid, corticosteroids, and maybe antibiotics, an enteral feeding tube is sometimes added to supplement eating. Alternatively, and often because an intravenous line is already in place, parenteral nutrition support is used in this situation. Either way, the nutrition is given primarily to support the child while the medical treatment is taking effect. Sometimes the child also receives nutrition support before surgery to improve wound healing. (Wound healing is sometimes impaired in a child with a poor nutritional state.)

Crohn's Disease

Drug treatment is not the only approach to improving the symptoms of Crohn's disease. Using specialized liquid formulas as the only source of nutrition for periods of six to eight weeks can reduce intestinal inflammation and digestive symptoms in some children with this disease (see chapter 10). Remission rates similar to rates with prednisone have been reported with formulas. Some studies have also found that children who receive ongoing formula may have fewer relapses. Because of limited data, the long-term benefit of diet treatment over drug treatment is unclear.

The major advantage of parenteral and enteral nutrition, as opposed to corticosteroids, is that the child has less exposure to prednisone. Prednisone will inhibit growth and cause bone weakness, both of which are complications that can cause long-term problems.

Nutrition support can also treat fistulas and obstructions, although they often recur when the treatment stops. If complications recur, then treatment with medications, surgery, or both are preferable to nutritional treatment.

For a child to make normal gains in weight and growth, disease activity must be controlled, and nutritional intake must be adequate for a long time—until the growth of the skeleton is complete. Over the course of the disease, children may need many changes in treatment, including medications, feeding support, and bowel surgery.

▣ 14

Complementary and Alternative Therapies

Although conventional medical therapy for Crohn's disease and ulcerative colitis has greatly improved over the last twenty-five years, it is still far from perfect. Medications commonly used to treat IBD may have unpleasant side effects for some children. In addition, many of our most effective medications (immunomodulators and biologics) reduce the activity of the immune system and therefore may increase the risk of infection or lymphoma. Nutritional therapy, though safe, often requires children to stop eating and to drink formulas that don't taste very good. Because IBD is a serious illness, currently without perfect treatments or a cure, many patients investigate complementary and alternative medicine (CAM).

The U.S. National Center for Complementary and Integrative Health (NCCIH) describes *alternative medicine* as the use of nonmainstream products and practices *in place of* conventional medicine. *Complementary medicine* refers to using nonmainstream approaches *with* conventional treatment. The concept of *integrative medicine* attempts to bring conventional (mainstream) and complementary approaches together in a coordinated way, with an emphasis on the importance of nutrition, exercise, stress management, and a strong support network. CAM treatments include dietary supplements, megadose vitamins, massage therapy, acupuncture, magnet therapy, meditation, yoga, energy-based therapies such as therapeutic touch, and spiritual healing. While standard medical approaches go through a long and careful research process to prove they are safe and effective, CAM therapies do not, so information about the effectiveness of CAM treatments is less reliable.

Surveys taken over the past several years show that about half of all children and adults with IBD seek CAM treatments. Most likely, those who seek CAM treatments are people who are not responding well to conventional treatments. Doctors want what is best for their patients, but most have not received formal training in the use of CAM. Thus, given the lack of good data and provider experience with nontraditional approaches, patients and their families often find their physicians reluctant to recommend specific CAM treatments or, in some cases, to even discuss them. The result is that many patients learn about such therapies from friends, acquaintances, and increasingly from social networks and other Internet-based resources. To date, there is not enough evidence to recommend CAM therapies routinely. Nevertheless, in this chapter we review some of the complementary treatments used for IBD (table 14.1).

Table 14.1
Complementary and alternative medicine (CAM) that can be used in addition to traditional IBD therapies

Herbs and botanicals	*Diet and nutritional therapy*
Curcumin	Low FODMAP diet
Aloe vera	Semi-vegetarian diet
Wormwood	Specific carbohydrate diet (SCD)
Boswellia serrata	*Mind-body practices*
Wheatgrass	Deep breathing
Nonherbal pharmaceuticals	Biofeedback
Low-dose naltrexone	Guided imagery
Omega-3 fatty acids	Hypnotherapy
Glucosamine/chondroitin	Meditation
Microbiota manipulations	Yoga
Probiotics	Tai chi
Fecal microbiota transplantation	Qigong
Whipworm eggs	Acupuncture
	Moxibustion
	Acupressure
	Massage
	Music therapy

General Information about CAM

Weighing Risks and Benefits

When considering any therapy, including CAM, it is important to weigh the risks and benefits. Unfortunately, very little high-quality data have been published on the safety and effectiveness of CAM in IBD. This is largely because of the tremendous expense of conducting well-designed scientific studies.

On the positive side, the medical and patient community has shown increasing interest in understanding the potential role of CAM therapies in the management of IBD. But the reality is that most CAM studies in IBD have been low quality. The current evidence is mostly anecdotal, meaning based on personal testimony or case reports rather than objective measurements, or from studies on small numbers of patients, with unclear and inconsistent definitions of response and remission, not based on the more vigorous definitions expected by academic medical publications. Responses often focus on an aspect or symptom that improved, a sense of feeling better, without objective assessments, such as complete normalization of symptoms, absence of signs of inflammation in lab tests, or, importantly, endoscopic mucosal healing (healing in the intestinal lining confirmed by endoscopy examination; see chapter 9).

In recent years, however, scientific studies of CAM therapies have been increasing. Clinical trials (controlled studies with measurable data) are providing some evidence on the safety and effectiveness of individual CAM therapies. Data from these trials allow doctors to feel more confident in recommending specific interventions and integrating CAM into conventional medical care.

When considering CAM, it is important to identify the goal of the therapy or intervention. For example, is the goal to turn off intestinal inflammation or to address specific symptoms such as joint pain, mouth ulcers, diarrhea, constipation, bloating, abdominal pain, appetite, lack of energy or fatigue, general sense of well-being, or symptoms of irritable bowel syndrome (IBS)? As emphasized elsewhere in this book, symptom control is not the same thing as adequate disease control.

To be sure, feeling well is important, but there can be a disconnect between feeling well and having sufficient control of inflammation. This is particularly true when considering the effects of major changes to a person's diet. It is possible to feel great yet still have significant inflammation—even if inflammation markers in lab tests are improving or normal. In children and teenagers, continued good growth and development are also crucial signs to track because lack of good growth may be the only sign of ongoing significant inflammation in a child who otherwise has no symptoms or abnormal lab results.

Understanding Products Used in CAM

Often the specific herbs, fish oil, probiotic, or other CAM therapy used in a clinical trial is not commercially available or readily accessible. Thus, the wormwood or curcumin preparations used in a study that suggested benefit in German and Japanese populations is not likely to be the same wormwood or curcumin formulations that you can pick up at a local pharmacy or farmers' market. For herbs, the specific part of the plant that is used and where and how it is grown can affect the desired properties, potency, and dosing. Additionally, CAM products tend not to be well regulated. They are not subject to the same strict, detailed labeling standards of prescription medications. This makes it difficult to compare products and determine effective dosing.

An essential point to understand when evaluating CAM products is that not everything "natural" is safe. Tobacco is natural, yet cigarette smoking is linked not only with lung cancer but, in CD, with worsened disease. Some herbs may contain natural steroids, but corticosteroids, whether natural or pharmaceutical, can have undesirable effects.

Another important distinction to recognize is that something touted as being "anti-inflammatory" does not necessarily have an anti-inflammatory effect on the *gastrointestinal tract*. For example, ibuprofen and other non-steroidal anti-inflammatory drugs reduce inflammation in the joints and other areas of the body, but they irritate and cause inflammation in the stomach and intestines and can worsen IBD; the same may be true of some anti-inflammatory herbs.

Some products (such as megavitamins) cause stomach or intestinal upset and other side effects. Others have been found to contain contaminants such as toxic amounts of heavy metals (e.g., mercury, arsenic, lead), as well as even some amounts of human placenta! Among alternative remedies and supplements (and their contaminants), some cause liver or kidney damage, while others may be laced with prescription drugs (such as corticosteroids) or even street drugs (such as "ecstasy").

Keep in mind that herbs being sold as treatments for IBD, or for some aspect of it, are delivered at pharmaceutical doses, sometimes for an extended length of time. Some products, even though homeopathic, may unexpectedly make IBD worse. Other supplements have blood-thinning properties or may alter how the body metabolizes prescribed medications (referred to as herb-drug interactions). For those taking multiple supplements, herb-herb interactions are another potential risk.

Although good information on herbal supplements can be found on the Internet, the available information may be incomplete or not applicable to your child's specific situation. There is also a lot of bad information, misinformation, and hype. Therefore, it is important to discuss supplement use with your child's doctor.

Having Realistic Expectations

Compared to corticosteroids or biologic therapies, CAM therapies often take much longer to demonstrate their full potential benefits. Although some CAM treatments might be used to quiet down a flare, others may have the best chance of working once the inflammation has been reduced with medication, as part of a longer-term maintenance strategy, or to prevent symptom or disease recurrence after surgery, when many children with IBD start with a "clean slate."

The key to many medical treatments, particularly long-term approaches, is *adherence*, which means following through with the therapy as directed. Adherence can be challenging with increasingly complex regimens, multiple supplements, and restrictive diets, especially if the treatments require a long-term commitment. All patients, including children, have a tendency to stray from their recommended therapy plans, especially once they start to feel better. Not adhering to the prescribed therapies is one of the most common reasons for an IBD flare. Importantly, symptoms may not return immediately; they may start weeks to months after stopping a therapy.

Most complementary health approaches fall into one of two broad subgroups—natural products or mind and body practices. While both traditional and alternative paths can work to varying degrees, sometimes really well, in many instances, a single intervention is unlikely to achieve optimal long-lasting wellness on its own.

Herbs and Botanicals

Plants have been used for medicinal purposes for centuries around the world. Sometimes a single pure herb is used, while other preparations may contain a variety of potentially effective ingredients to address one or more symptoms. The healing components of many plants have been identified. Some possess anti-inflammatory, antioxidant, antibacterial, antifungal, antispasmodic, stimulant, sedative, anticancer, or immune properties. Some, like aspirin and morphine, have been adopted into standard medical practice.

The medicinal component of a plant may be found in its berries, or in other plants, the leaves, stems, stalks, bark, roots, seeds, nuts, or flowers. Herbal supplements may come in the form of teas, pills, powders, oils, syrups, juices, creams, lotions, or compresses. The same plant grown in different regions may have different properties. So when looking for the "right" product for your child, it is important to know whether the product contains the therapeutic component of the plant and to understand that the dose of the active ingredient can vary among products. Possible effects on IBD have been identified for some herbs. Although most experiences with herbs in IBD are from personal testimony, small studies, primarily in adults, have been done, typically in countries outside the United States (see below). For nearly all herbal products studied, larger and longer-term clinical trials are needed to determine how safe they are, and how well they work, in IBD.

Curcumin

The yellow pigment in the spice turmeric, called *curcumin*, has anti-inflammatory properties supported by measurable evidence from clinical trials and studies in animals with intestinal inflammation similar to IBD. In a small four-week study of adults with mildly to moderately active UC, 3 grams of curcumin a day when added to mesalamine was associated with clinical remission and even endoscopic healing of the intestinal lining compared to the effects of a placebo (inactive substance, like a sugar pill) added to mesalamine. Another study suggested that 1 gram of curcumin twice a day when added to "standard" medicines helped maintain remission in adults with UC over a six-month period. On the other hand, when curcumin enemas were studied, they seemed to have no significant effect in people with mild to moderate inflammation of the rectum and sigmoid colon. Small studies in CD suggest some potential benefit.

Aloe Vera

Aloe vera has been used medicinally for more than five thousand years and is thought to have several compounds that can affect processes in the body. Aloe vera gel at a dose of 100 ml twice a day was given to adults with mildly to moderately active UC in England. After four weeks, the symptoms of UC improved in those taking the aloe compared with placebo; however, no significant differences were seen in laboratory results and no healing of the intestinal lining was noted. Aloe can have a laxative effect and cause diarrhea.

Wormwood

Wormwood *(Artemisia absinthium)* is a wild plant of the daisy family with anti-inflammatory and immunosuppressive properties. Wormwood or placebo was added to the treatment regimens of adults with active CD in a six-week study in Germany. The adults receiving wormwood showed significant decrease in CD symptoms and depression, as well as an increase in quality of life compared with the group that received the placebo. In another study, patients with CD on steroids treated for ten weeks with an herbal blend containing wormwood showed improved symptoms compared with the placebo group during the five-month study periods.

Boswellia serrata (Indian frankincense)

Boswellia serrata (Indian frankincense) has anti-inflammatory properties. When given to adults with active colitis at a dose of 300 mg three times a day for six weeks, *Boswellia serrata* seemed to work as well as 5-ASA medication. In another study, done over a two-month period, *Boswellia serrata* appeared to work just as well as a 5-ASA drug in improving symptoms of CD. However, a different study showed no improvement in using *Boswellia serrata* as maintenance therapy for CD patients in clinical remission — in fact, this study had to be ended early because the group receiving this herb was doing no better than the group receiving placebo.

Wheatgrass

The young wheat plant harvested prior to the formation of the flower head, called wheatgrass (*Triticum aestivum*), has been shown to have antioxidant and anti-inflammatory properties. Wheatgrass juice was studied in adults with active UC in Israel. Participants drank 100 cc (about 3.3 ounces) of wheatgrass juice or placebo daily for four weeks. Wheatgrass juice was associated with improved symptoms and decreased rectal bleeding.

Other Herbs and Botanicals

Some additional studies of mild to moderate UC have shown improvement in symptoms with other herbs and botanicals, including *Andrographis paniculata* extract, *Plantago ovata* (psyllium) seeds, germinated barley, and silymarin (extracted from milk thistle).

Nonherbal Pharmaceuticals

Low-Dose Naltrexone

Low-dose naltrexone (LDN) has been proposed as a possible therapy for IBD. A small study in children with moderate to severe Crohn's disease suggested LDN taken for eight to sixteen weeks could improve symptoms and quality of life compared with placebo; however, the researchers did not perform endoscopy to see if the lining of the intestines showed healing. In a small study of adults with active CD, most of those receiving LDN for twelve weeks experienced symptom improvement—30 percent even achieved clinical remission. Compared with those taking placebo, however, the patients on LDN did not show improved healing of the intestines. Thus, published data on LDN as a therapy for IBD are still quite limited. LDN's potential side effects include nausea, headache, dizziness, anxiety, fatigue, vivid dreams, and sleep disturbances.

Omega-3 Fatty Acids

Omega-3 fatty acids, such as those found in fish oil, have anti-inflammatory properties. A one-year Italian study found that pediatric patients with Crohn's disease who were in remission were less likely to flare when supplemented with fish oil in addition to 5-ASA therapy. Larger studies done later, however, have failed to confirm benefits for maintenance of remission. There is little information about fish oils in UC. Omega-3 fatty acids appear to be safe, though they may cause diarrhea or upper GI tract symptoms, and high doses of fish oil can increase bleeding risk, increase levels of low-density lipoprotein (LDL, or "bad" cholesterol), and cause problems with controlling blood sugar.

Glucosamine and Chondroitin

Glucosamine, a dietary supplement, is often taken with chondroitin to help with joint pain and swelling, which may be experienced by some people who have IBD. Doctors often recommend avoiding or limiting NSAIDs (nonsteroidal anti-inflammatory drugs) such as ibuprofen, because they may worsen IBD. Studies looking at glucosamine and chondroitin are mixed, and though not specifically studied in IBD, these supplements may provide some relief. Glucosamine supplements are typically made from the skeletons of shellfish; chondroitin, from cow or shark cartilage. Research suggests that glucosamine and chondroitin don't appear to have a lot of risks. Some individuals find turmeric and fish oil help with IBD-associated joint pain.

Manipulation of the Intestine Microbiota

As mentioned in chapter 2, the trillions of bacteria and other living organisms in our intestinal tract (called the *microbiota* or *microbiome*) may play a role in the development of IBD or in triggering IBD flares.

Probiotics

Probiotics (good bacteria) may provide some benefits to health. The compounds commonly used in treatment are made of bacteria, such as *Lactobacillus* and *Bifidobacterium* species, that populate the intestinal tract and generally do not cause disease. Several probiotic preparations are available in supermarkets, health food stores, and over the Internet. Improving the balance of good versus bad bacteria may aid in digestion, help protect the intestine from harmful bacteria, promote a healthier immune system, and reduce intestinal inflammation. Small studies in UC suggest possible benefit, especially for pouchitis. Studies of various probiotics in the treatment of CD have not demonstrated clear benefit. Large, well-done, longer-term studies are lacking. So the role of probiotics in IBD remains controversial but continues to be a topic of ongoing interest and research. Probiotics may help prevent relapses of *Clostridium difficile* infection, prevent antibiotic-associated diarrhea, and help reduce symptoms such as bloating. Probiotics are generally considered fairly safe, but their effectiveness in reducing inflammation in IBD remains unclear.

Fecal Microbiota Transplantation

Fecal microbiota transplantation (FMT), also referred to as stool or fecal transplant, is a very effective treatment for refractory or recurrent *Clostridium difficile* infections, but the role of FMT in IBD is not established. Many studies are in progress to address that question. FMT does not in reality "reestablish" one's own gut flora, but rather transplants the microbiota of another individual—a presumed healthy donor. While the concept is very interesting, and there is evidence suggesting potential benefit in some individuals, FMT is not currently an FDA-approved therapy for IBD. If used in IBD, it is likely that repeated dosing, perhaps from more than one individual, would be necessary for longer-term benefits. When properly performed, FMT seems generally safe in the short run, but it carries a risk of introducing infection and the possibility of causing an IBD flare. Informed consents for individuals electing to undergo FMT might also include the theoretical increased risk of developing a disease related to the donor, because foreign gut bacteria could trigger conditions that might not otherwise express themselves, including a tendency toward obesity, metabolic syndrome, irritable bowel syndrome, allergic disorders, neurologic disorders, or even other autoimmune conditions.

Whipworm Eggs

Data on whipworm eggs (*Trichuris suis* ova; TSO) as a therapy in IBD are limited. In a CD study, most participants who swallowed live TSO every three weeks for twenty-four weeks experienced symptom improvement, but healing of the intestines was not checked. The effects of TSO taken every two weeks for twelve weeks were tested in adults with UC, and although some people had improvement in their symptoms, the TSO was really no better than placebo.

Diet and Nutritional Therapy

As discussed in chapters 10 and 13, nutritional therapy can play a significant role in treating IBD. Some nutritional interventions help with symptoms. Others can influence inflammation. Food components may directly irritate the intestines, alter the microbiota (bacteria, viral, and fungal), or work via *epigenetic* mechanisms, which "turn off" or "turn on" genes, through interactions with the gut environment.

Numerous studies have shown that dramatic diet changes (formula or real food) can lead to shifts in the gut microbiota in days to weeks. Other lifestyle choices shown to affect the gut microbiota include smoking, smoking cessation, stress, and exercise. There is, however, a tendency for the microbiota to revert toward its initial composition (often along with return of symptoms) within two weeks of resuming one's usual diet, old habits, and lifestyle.

While nutritional formula therapies are safe and nutritionally sound, for them to work as actual therapy to treat IBD, your child would have to stop eating most regular food and mainly drink formulas (see chapter 10). Drinking formulas doesn't always taste very good and can get boring, especially if done for long periods. Real-food diets, especially if done in conjunction with other positive lifestyle modifications, can also alter the gut microbiota as well as improve symptoms and potentially even disease activity. The three real-food diets gaining popularity as complementary therapies in the IBD patient community are the low FODMAP diet, the semi-vegetarian diet, and the specific carbohydrate diet. In general the study of real-food (also called whole-food) diets is an active area of research.

Low FODMAP Diet

The low FODMAP diet limits certain types of fermentable sugars that may be poorly digested and absorbed. While more commonly used to reduce symptoms of irritable bowel syndrome, a small study found that patients with IBD experienced improvement in symptoms of diarrhea, abdominal pain, and bloating while on the diet. This diet is not generally intended for long-term use but rather to eliminate symptoms and identify symptom-producing foods.

Semi-vegetarian Diet

Preliminary data suggest that a semi-vegetarian diet (SVD) may reduce the chances of an IBD flare. The role of an SVD as a maintenance therapy was explored in a small CD study in Japan. All adults entered the study in clinical remission and continued on 5-ASA therapy. Seventy-five percent of those who continued their usual diets experienced a flare. On the other hand, 92 percent of those who ate a long-term SVD during the two-year study successfully remained in clinical remission.

Specific Carbohydrate Diet

The specific carbohydrate diet (SCD) is a real-food, gluten-free, grain-free diet that limits dairy, avoids processed foods and starches, and allows no additional sugar beyond those naturally found in fruits, vegetables, and honey. It is probably the most commonly attempted diet for IBD. The diet was originally designed by Dr. Sidney Haas as a treatment for celiac disease, before gluten was discovered to be the culprit in that condition. The diet was then promoted for IBD by Elaine Gottschall, whose daughter had been very sick with UC and achieved clinical remission with the SCD while under Dr. Haas's care. The SCD diet has not been well studied, but personal testimonies and small studies suggest potential benefit for some, including improvement or resolution of symptoms and improvement in tests of inflammation.

The SCD involves an introductory elimination phase followed by gradual introduction of "SCD-legal" foods, while completely avoiding "SCD-illegal" foods and products. The SCD diet is hard to do properly. Sticking to the diet rigorously is important, but that can be very difficult to do. Initial weight loss in the range of 5–15 pounds is often observed. There is a risk of certain vitamin and mineral deficiencies in those pursuing the diet as part of a longer-term strategy, so it is best to work with a dietician familiar with SCD to optimize the chances of success, while ensuring adequate nutrition for well-being, healing, and growth.

Such diets, especially those practiced long term, are not for everyone and require lots of motivation and planning. They are not just diets but huge lifestyle commitments. These can be done in a medically and nutritionally sound way under the supervision of a doctor and a dietician. Again, it is important to remember that there can be a disconnect between feeling well and achieving adequate disease control. With dietary manipulations, your child might feel better, even well, and her inflammation markers might improve or normalize, but there can still be significant ongoing inflammation. Periodic endoscopic evaluation is crucial to make sure the strategy is working well enough. Failure to recognize inflammation can lead to disease complications, including fistulas, perforations, strictures, and poor growth, sometimes even resulting in the need for surgery.

Lifestyle Modification

A good night's sleep helps maintain physical and mental health, and it can improve energy, concentration, and immune function. The artificial light emitted by the screens of electronic devices (phone, tablet, computer, TV) adversely affects sleep quality and suppresses melatonin, the hormone that signals the body that it's time to sleep. Studies show that stopping screen time 2 hours before bedtime improves sleep quality.

Exercise has many health benefits, yet only 1 out of 4 children gets enough exercise each day. Between video games, TV, online social networking, and homework, children and teens (and adults) are becoming increasingly sedentary. Exercise has been shown to have numerous positive effects, including (1) promoting healthy muscles and bones; (2) decreasing stress; (3) increasing energy; (4) encouraging social interaction; (5) helping with relaxation; (6) improving sleep; and (7) shifting the gut microbiota to help calm an overactive immune system.

Mindfulness-Based Interventions

Many people with IBD, including children, feel that stress affects their disease. Stress induces a cascade of effects that can create inflammation, impair healing, and suppress the immune system, increasing susceptibility to colds, flu, and other infections. When faced with a danger, the fight-or-flight response automatically kicks in, increasing the heart rate and blood flow to muscles, diverting blood flow from the intestines and other less vital areas. While such a response can be crucial for life-threatening situations, most of us fortunately don't face those daily. Smaller stressors, however, *even perceived potential stresses*, can trigger the same responses, increasing adrenaline and heart rate day after day, over time hardwiring the established responses. Negative effects on the body can be cumulative.

No one can avoid stress altogether, but your child can learn to manage the stress response. Mindfulness-based interventions lead to increased awareness of muscle tension and other physical sensations of stress. Your child can then make a conscious effort to start relaxation techniques at the first sensation, preventing stress from spiraling out of control. With practice the brain can be retrained to create different stress response pathways and new relaxation pathways, changing what's happening in the body. A study investigating the effects of relaxation training in patients with IBD found significant improvements in pain, anxiety, depression, mood, stress, and quality of life, including bowel symptoms, within the relaxation group, but not in the usual-care group.

Although not all mind-body practices described below have been specifically studied in IBD, they provide techniques that can help your child focus on the present moment, calm his brain, and slow his heart rate and breathing, providing effective tools in addressing stress and optimizing health and wellness.

Deep Breathing

Deep, or relaxed, breathing focuses on deep, slow, smooth, even-paced breathing using the diaphragm to expand the lungs. Slower, deeper breathing reduces heart rate and blood pressure; releases endorphins, the body's natural painkillers; and can help reduce anxiety and stress.

Biofeedback

Biofeedback is a technique that uses electrical sensors to provide information about the body through visual or audible feedback. Using that feedback, your child can learn to use her thoughts to control various bodily functions. Breathing sensors can help her learn to control her breathing more consciously. A pulse sensor placed on the fingertip or earlobe measures increases and decreases in heart rate. Temperature or thermal sensors attached to the fingers measure skin temperature and blood flow to the skin. EMG (electromyography) biofeedback provides information about muscle tension. Under stress, heart and breathing rates increase, and blood vessels clamp down. By recognizing these signals early in the stress response cycle, your child can learn how to proactively use the power of thought to induce positive physical changes on her own by controlling her breathing, heart rate, blood pressure, skin temperature, and muscle tension to relax. Though the initial awareness and feedback comes from the sensors, with training and practice, she can learn to eventually recognize these subtle changes and counteract them without the help of technology. Biofeedback can be used to help manage stress, anxiety, headaches and other chronic pain, constipation, incontinence, IBS symptoms, and medication side effects.

Guided Imagery

Guided imagery, also referred to as visualization, involves creating specific mental images to produce desired responses in the body: physical, emotional, or spiritual. The created images and sensations don't just stay in the mind; they are passed on to produce measurable changes in a wide range of bodily functions, including heart and breathing rates, blood pressure, and even immune function. Research using PET (positron emission tomography) scan imaging has shown that imagining something activates the same parts of the brain as actually experiencing it does.

The steps in guided imagery involve finding a quiet, comfortable place and position to relax. The mind is cleared of all chatter, worries, and distractions by focusing attention on breathing, with emphasis on taking slow, deep breaths and releasing all random thoughts during exhalation. A desired image or intention is then incorporated and focused on. A positive message or affirmation or feeling can be coupled with the image to be stored within the brain for easy recall at a later time. If certain images bring your child feelings of peace, they can be incorporated into his daily surroundings, such as a picture on the home screen of a computer or phone.

With practice, your child can learn to practice guided imagery on his own, but early on, it is often helpful to be guided in a one-on-one, small group setting, or by a CD or digital audio file that contains guided imagery coaching by someone experienced. This technique has been used to help induce relaxation, cope with stress and depression, reduce anxiety before surgery, help with nausea, reduce the frequency of migraine headaches, and decrease the need for pain medication.

Hypnotherapy

Hypnotherapy, also called hypnosis or hypnotic suggestion, is usually guided by a therapist who uses verbal repetition and mental images to help achieve a trance-like state in which the person usually feels calm and relaxed and experiences heightened focus and concentration, a state in which the mind is more open to suggestions. After the hypnosis session, once returned to a normal state of consciousness, individuals then practice the suggested behavior. Hypnotherapy has been shown to help people learn to cope better with anxiety, stress, and pain, as well as to help change behaviors, such as smoking. While the mechanism remains unclear, measurable changes in even immune response have been observed.

Meditation

Meditation refers to a group of techniques that help clear and calm the mind from the stream of thoughts that normally occupies it, by focusing attention on breathing or a word, phrase, or sound to create a state of physical relaxation, mental calmness, and psychological balance. Potential benefits include increased self-awareness, improved focus on the present moment, reduced negative emotions, improved memory and concentration, as well as enhanced ability to manage tension, anxiety, depression, headaches, sleep problems, nausea, vomiting, and pain. Meditation is simple, inexpensive, and can be practiced by anyone. There is no one right way to meditate. There are many styles of meditation:

Breath meditation involves a focus on breathing that is deep, slow, and smooth, consciously observing each inhalation and exhalation.

Mindfulness meditation focuses on bringing all attention to increased awareness and acceptance of the present moment by experiencing it without reacting to it or making any judgments about it.

Transcendental meditation uses a mantra in the form of a sound, word, or phrase that is repeated over and over, either out loud or silently, to focus or hold attention with the goal of keeping distracting thoughts out of conscious awareness.

Body scanning involves sequentially focusing attention on individual parts of the body to become aware of the various sensations, including pain, tension, and relaxation. This can be combined with breathing and relaxation techniques.

Progressive muscle relaxation focuses on the slow, steady contraction or tensing of a muscle, followed by a gradual relaxation of that muscle to identify areas where stress is stored, then deliberately relieve that tension. The process is then repeated on other groups of muscles in succession to reach a state of deep relaxation.

Guided meditation, similar to guided imagery, uses mental images of places or situations to create a relaxed state. It may incorporate relaxing or inspiring music, sounds, sights, smells, and textures. Guiding may be done in a group setting or alone and can be facilitated using a recorded audio program or script.

Moving meditation practices, such as walking meditation, yoga, tai chi, and qigong, follow the same general principles of meditation but add movement to the mix.

Walking meditation focuses not on the destination but on the subtle movements used during walking and on feeling the earth beneath the feet. The pace is slowed down and attention is focused on each movement of the legs and feet, on the lifting, moving, and placing of each foot on the ground while moving forward. This can be practiced anywhere.

Mind-Body Practices

Yoga, tai chi, and qigong are mind-body practices that can be performed alone or in a group setting. They create a peaceful feeling while teaching balance, enhancing flexibility and endurance, and building muscle strength. These practices may help your child manage stress, anxiety, and depression; improve mood, energy, and stamina; and potentially improve concentration and memory. They have been shown to lower blood pressure, help relieve chronic pain, benefit those with sleeping difficulties, and potentially have a positive effect on arthritis and on bone health.

Yoga involves a series of yoga postures with each specific pose
connected to breathing—exhaling during certain movements and
inhaling with others. There are different forms of yoga. Power
yoga is a vigorous freestyle form. Hatha yoga, on the other hand,
tends to be a slower-paced, more relaxed style, making it great
yoga for beginners or those looking to hold poses longer. Hatha
yoga is the general category that encompasses most of the styles
practiced in Western societies. Yoga is fairly simple to learn. The
ultimate goal is to reach complete peacefulness of mind and body.

Tai chi, originally developed for self-defense, involves a series of
movements performed in a slow, focused manner, accompanied
by deep breathing. Each posture flows into the next without
pause, ensuring that the body is in constant motion.

Qigong is a form of meditative exercise in which slow, smooth, fluid,
and rhythmic movements are coordinated with controlled
breathing to improve the flow of energy, or qi.

Traditional Chinese Practices

Practitioners of traditional Chinese medicine believe that blockages in the
flow of qi lead to imbalances that manifest as disease. Acupuncture, moxibustion, and acupressure aim to remove blockages in the flow of qi, the
vital energy or life force, that flows through pathways in the body (called
meridians) to regulate physical, emotional, mental, and spiritual health.

Acupuncture involves the strategic insertion of very thin needles
through the skin's surface into specific points along the body's
meridians to reestablish the flow of qi, restoring balance and
health. Acupuncture needles are much thinner than a needle
used to draw blood, and they have a beveled tip, so they push the
tissue to the side instead of cutting it. They are typically not
inserted deeply. Acupuncture is often performed in a relaxed
setting, with the individual sitting or lying on a special table. The
practitioner places five to twenty needles, which are left in place

for 15 to 20 minutes or so. The World Health Organization recognizes acupuncture as a potentially effective therapy for a variety of medical conditions, including nausea, constipation, abdominal pain, anxiety, headaches, neck and back pain, and menstrual problems. Acupuncture is usually a component of a broader treatment program.

Moxibustion is a traditional Chinese medicinal practice of heat therapy that uses burning moxa made from dried mugwort (*Artemisia argyi*) to warm specific regions and meridian points with the intention of stimulating the flow of qi. Practitioners burn the moxa on or very near the surface of the skin, sometimes on acupuncture needles, to achieve the desired effect. Studies in IBD have been vigorously done, and some suggest potential benefit in disease activity and quality of life.

Acupressure, sometimes referred to as *shiatsu*, involves applying physical pressure to specific points on the surface of the body using a finger, hand, elbow, or device to restore the flow of qi. Acupressure can be used for relaxation or to help with nausea, constipation, diarrhea, headache, musculoskeletal pain and tension, depression, anxiety, and sleep difficulties.

Massage

Massage, considered one of the oldest healing arts, is a general term for pressing, rubbing, and manipulating the skin, muscles, tendons, and ligaments, sometimes with specific health goals in mind. There are many different kinds of massage, including the popular Swedish massage, as well as sports, deep tissue, and trigger point massage. The practice increases blood flow through the body; releases endorphins, the body's natural painkillers; and decreases some of the chemicals associated with stress, like cortisol. The power of human touch and the ambience, which often includes a quiet setting with relaxing music and sometimes aromatherapy, may also play a role in the healing power of massage. Studies have shown that massage may be helpful for anxiety, stress, insomnia, digestive disorders, muscle tension, fibromyalgia, headaches, and various other types of pain.

Music Therapy

In music therapy, qualified music therapists use various music interventions (listening to, moving to, singing, and/or creating) to address an individual's physical needs. Music therapy may be used to reduce anxiety, help manage pain, improve functioning and well-being, and enhance quality of life.

Aromatherapy

Aromatherapy is the therapeutic use of essential oils extracted from the roots, leaves, seeds, or blossoms of plants to encourage psychological and physical well-being.

Complementary practices offer additional options to address the wide range of symptoms experienced by children with IBD. Some therapies may help with disease control or specific symptoms; others may improve day-to-day functioning and overall well-being.

When looking for CAM practitioners, it is important to take the same steps as when choosing a doctor. Check practitioners' training and credentials. Specifically ask about their experience with IBD *especially with children* (and be aware that alternative care practitioners may confuse IBS with IBD). Ask about the likelihood of response, time to response, potential side effects, anticipated cost and duration of treatment, and whether the therapy is covered by insurance.

Individuals and families considering any of the CAM approaches should discuss them with their IBD doctor and use CAM to complement prescribed therapies, not in place of doctor-recommended treatments. Just as with traditional medicine, not everyone responds in the same way to CAM. Most CAM practices are not stand-alone interventions. Rather, the better results are likely to be achieved when used in addition to traditional IBD therapies.

Part IV
Living with IBD

▣ 15

Family Life

A child's chronic illness affects the whole family, and each family member influences the child with IBD. In this chapter, we discuss the concerns of parents and siblings of children with IBD who have been identified in focus group research. (Focus group research involves extensive interviews of many people by professional researchers who attempt to identify what these people have in common. In this case, researchers interviewed families who had a child with a chronic disease.) We also look at the family as a whole and discuss what we know about what helps families cope effectively when a child has a chronic illness. (Chapter 16 offers insight into how children cope with chronic disease at different stages of development.)

Parents' Concerns

In focus group research, the concern mentioned most often by parents involves how IBD will affect their child's future. Will their child be able to participate in sports and the social activities that are so important to teenagers? Will his growth rate and entrance into puberty catch up to his friends? What will happen if she goes away to college? How will he manage dating and finding a significant other? What about having children of her own? Will IBD affect career opportunities?

As adults, parents can see the possible broader implications of having IBD. The unknown is always difficult, but it may be reassuring to know that according to research, people with IBD typically have the same levels of educational and occupational success as the general population.

Young children do not have the capacity to understand the long-term implications of their condition. They are more concerned with the immediate future (today or tomorrow). When children are unsure about a situation, they often look to their parents to determine how they should react. As a parent, you can communicate important information about IBD to your young child in a matter-of-fact manner, using simple terms. Keeping a straightforward "This may be tough, but we can handle it" attitude will help your child maintain this attitude, too. Don't worry if your child seems more concerned about day-to-day activities than any long-term difficulties associated with having IBD. This is normal behavior for young children and does not mean that your child has a problem with accepting the facts of the disease.

As children reach the teen years, they begin to understand the possible broader long-term implications of having IBD, and they may express concerns they have not mentioned before. Follow your child's cues when it comes to answering questions, giving advice, or simply listening and sympathizing. You may want to suggest that your teen discuss these issues with her doctor, with or without you in the room. Your teen would also benefit from getting to know other teens with IBD. As with the young child, the matter-of-fact "This may be tough, but we can handle it" attitude goes a long way in helping your teen cope with IBD.

Another concern often mentioned by parents in focus groups involves school. Issues may include bathroom access, make-up work when the child is absent, taking medications at school, educating school personnel about IBD, and concerns about classmates' and school personnel's sensitivity to the child's needs (see chapter 18).

Additional concerns identified in focus group research include side effects of medications (see chapter 10) and struggling with feelings of guilt. Did I give my child IBD? Why didn't I take her stomachaches more seriously sooner? Am I a good parent?

Many of the symptoms of IBD are not specific and could occur in any number of health conditions. Therefore, there is often a delay in diagnosis. Some research suggests that children experience IBD symptoms for an average of ten months before being diagnosed with IBD. Even pediatric gastroenterologists, who specialize in children's digestive diseases, don't assume that their own children's abdominal pain and diarrhea mean they have IBD.

All parents struggle with concerns about being a good parent. Parents of children with special needs (such as a chronic illness) may struggle with these concerns more than the typical parent does. Research has shown that children do best with parents who balance nurturing with appropriate expectations about behavior (and discipline), regardless of whether the child has a chronic illness. There is a wide range of good parenting behaviors, and what you do in the long run, consistently, is most important. Having a child with IBD means that you may face challenges that other parents do not, but otherwise, parenting a child with IBD is no different from parenting any other child.

Siblings' Concerns

In focus group research, the primary concern of siblings was feeling like they were kept in the dark about IBD. Prior to diagnosis, they may have known their brother or sister was ill, but they may not have been told about doctor visits and procedures. Many siblings are taught about IBD during the initial diagnosis and education phase but are less informed about the later course of their sibling's disease. Siblings want to know this information, and they usually have practical questions about IBD: Is it contagious? Is it fatal? Does it hurt? What kinds of medicine will my brother or sister have to take? For how long?

In addition, siblings are often put in the role of a reporter, as family friends and school personnel ask them about their sibling with IBD. Parents can make sure all their children have the information they need and give them examples of things they can tell others who ask about their sibling.

Siblings may also feel that the child with IBD is favored or receives more of their parents' attention. They may view clinic visits as special times with Mom or Dad, especially if Mom and Dad combine clinic visits with a fun activity such as going out to eat. These concerns can be addressed in two ways. First, parents can engage in special one-on-one activities with each child, not just with the child who has IBD. Children love one-on-one attention from parents. Activities can include playing board games, helping with cooking, riding bikes together, reading aloud together, or working on a special project.

Second, parents should require all children, including the child with IBD, to follow all the usual family rules, live up to the same expectations, and share the same level of responsibility. The child with IBD can be expected to join in family recreational activities and to have the usual responsibilities and chores. Do not avoid disciplining the child with IBD, if discipline is necessary. Allowing a child with IBD to avoid responsibilities and discipline deprives the child of opportunities to learn how to cope with life—and with having IBD in the context of normal family life. It may also create problems with siblings, who may feel that the child with IBD is favored.

Family Concerns

Some families seem to take IBD and its challenges in stride. How do they do it? Researchers in other pediatric chronic illnesses have identified what helps families cope effectively. These families balance the demands of the illness with other family needs and responsibilities. Family life does not revolve around the illness. The illness must play a large role at times, but family life does not regularly center on it. These families also have clear boundaries and expectations. They maintain their usual family routines. They require all children, including the child with IBD, to follow all the usual rules, live up to the same expectations, and share the same level of responsibility, as well as receive consequences for inappropriate behavior.

Successful families have supportive social networks. Support systems, both formal and informal, can provide ongoing emotional support and the periodic practical support needed in managing clinic visits and hospitalizations. Such practical support may include transporting other children to and from school and activities. These families also have flexible family roles that can change as needed, and an open communication style that allows all family members to express feelings and needs.

In successful families, all family members, including siblings, have knowledge about the symptoms, treatment, and course of IBD. And they use active coping strategies. Active coping strategies include problem solving and actively seeking social support. Passive coping strategies include denial, avoidance, and withdrawal.

When to Seek Help

Since IBD affects the whole family, and since each family member affects the child with IBD, it is important to recognize when counseling would be helpful for any family member. Therapy with a psychologist, psychiatrist, or other mental health professional is a good idea any time behavioral or emotional problems significantly interfere with a person's performance in any area, such as school, work, social activities, or family relationships.

Specific warning signs of a problem that needs to be addressed with professional help include

- lowered grades
- lowered productivity at work
- significant absences (from school or work)
- social withdrawal
- lack of pleasure in social or recreational activities
- significant family stress in addition to IBD
- increased arguments with spouse, parents, or siblings

Mental health professionals who specialize in health psychology can help the child with IBD and other family members cope with the disease as well as its consequences. Taking medications on schedule, managing pain, feeling distress about medical procedures, and avoiding school—these and other stresses are often managed better with the help of a professional who can offer support as well as advice about practical things the child and family can do to help everyone cope.

▣ 16

Different Ages, Different Issues

Living with inflammatory bowel disease is not easy. It is a chronic condition, with unpredictable flares of symptoms that are difficult to manage. The symptoms include abdominal pain, bloody diarrhea, and low energy. In addition to the flares, long-term problems related to IBD include malnutrition, slow growth, and late puberty.

IBD may have an unpredictable course. Children may undergo invasive tests, complicated treatments, and sometimes surgery. All of this means that a diagnosis of IBD can be difficult to accept, particularly during childhood and adolescence. Most children and teens go through a period of adjusting, in both their emotions and their behavior, to a diagnosis of IBD. Many children experience periods of anger and even depression.

Several factors influence how a person reacts to having a chronic illness. How your child responds to IBD depends in part on his age, maturity level regarding cognition (thought processes), and the severity of the illness. Another factor in a child's reaction to the diagnosis is the parents' reaction. Parent-child conversations about IBD are essential, and they usually set the tone for the whole family. In this chapter, we discuss developmental landmarks—the differences in maturity and coping styles of children at different ages. This information will guide parents who are helping their child or teenager cope with IBD. Talking to your child in an age-appropriate and matter-of-fact way will help him cope with IBD and everything that goes along with having this disease. At times, it would be reasonable to seek help and guidance from mental health professionals like psychologists to help manage the new reality of a chronic disease, develop coping skills, and have screening for depression and anxiety. Our goal is to guide you to help your child live a fulfilling, productive life despite having a chronic illness.

Early Childhood: Ages 2 through 6

A child with IBD faces special issues that are connected to her developmental needs. Between 2 and 6 years of age, a child has many physical, emotional, and cognitive targets to reach. By reaching these targets, the child develops the independence, self-control, and language skills needed to begin school successfully.

Physically, the healthy preschooler grows more slowly than a baby. Parents notice that their child has less of an appetite than she had as an infant. A preschooler's eating habits can change noticeably from day to day. It can be difficult to tell the difference between normal appetite changes at this age and a reduced appetite from worsening IBD. Watch your child's growth carefully to make sure that the IBD is under control. Your child's doctor may need to order tests to help determine if IBD is making your child's appetite worse.

During early childhood, the main developmental work of the child includes

- improving self-control (for example, toilet training)
- learning a language
- getting used to separating from parents or other main caregivers

During the preschool years, language skills advance rapidly. Your child's vocabulary is growing noticeably, and sentences are more organized and complex. Preschoolers are also better at expressing their feelings and needs. Although children at this age may sound more adult, they see the world very differently from adults. For example, they might be afraid of monsters or have imaginary friends. It is normal for preschool children to express feelings of stress through behavior instead of words. Preschoolers are also fascinated with their bowel functioning.

In terms of cognitive growth, children in this age group often show both real-world concrete thinking (everything happens because of something I can see or touch) and magical thinking. Magical thinking means thinking that events in their lives happen because of their own thoughts, feelings, and behaviors; it also means mixing up cause and effect. While this view of the world is normal preschool behavior, it also affects how your child reacts to having IBD. Children may connect the symptoms of their disease with unrelated events or actions. Young children diagnosed with IBD often connect their symptoms (such as pain and diarrhea) with other events that happen at around the same time. For example, a 5-year-old might think that her bad behavior caused her IBD, and she may feel guilty.

The preschooler's magical view of the world can create challenges for her and for her parents when it is time for treatments or tests. Young children may have mistaken ideas about the reasons for procedures or hospitalizations. It is not uncommon for them to see such activities as a form of punishment rather than as being necessary for their care. In addition, they have difficulty understanding ideas such as amount and length of time (for example, "it will last only a short while" or "this will hurt only a little"). Parents often want to explain, "You need to have this blood test so the doctor can make you feel better." An explanation like this is usually not comforting at this age and can even add to the child's worry. The company of a calm, comforting parent is most important to the preschooler. Most children's hospitals have child-life specialists who can help children prepare for procedures, and they have a wealth of advice for parents.

Preschoolers often have a good idea of outside body parts, but inside body parts are still not real to them, and children connect them with many magical ideas.

Preschoolers worry about loss and about being left behind. These anxieties can complicate their reactions to medical stresses. They may be sad and angry about being separated from siblings during hospitalizations, or they may feel jealous about the good health of siblings, especially if the preschooler does not have the physical energy to take part in regular activities. Preschoolers who feel overwhelmed may behave like babies again (this is called *regression*), or they may lose skills they already learned (for example, toilet training).

You can help your young child with a new diagnosis of IBD by encouraging him to talk about the illness and by answering your child's questions in simple language that the child understands. Listen for elements of magical thinking that may be making your child nervous. Expect reactions such as "forgetting" about his illness during times of remission (when the disease is not active), or not showing distress even during IBD symptom flares. These reactions can be considered normal as long as your child cooperates with medical care and reaches all the right developmental benchmarks. Watch your child for changes in behavior or play. If you are concerned about your child's feelings, talk about your concerns with your child's pediatrician or pediatric gastroenterologist. They may have suggestions. It is often helpful to consult a mental health professional who specializes in helping children and parents adjust and cope.

Parents need to manage their own anxiety about the diagnosis and treatments of IBD. If you do not have a good support system, you need to put one in place. Talking things over with other adults, including other parents of children with IBD, and knowing you can call on them for logistical assistance if you need to will help you be available for your child. Finally, as mentioned in the previous chapter, it is critical to keep daily family life as normal as possible, including discipline. Your child needs to develop a self-image well beyond "being sick." Instead, your child should think of IBD as one of life's manageable challenges.

Middle Childhood: Ages 6 through 12

In middle childhood, children try hard to master their bodies and the environment. As children enter school, they become more independent and are more concerned about being accepted by their peers. Self-esteem is an important issue. In the child's mind, how she does in school, sports, and play are measures of how much she is "worth." She tries to master skills such as school behavior, sports, and special talents. A diagnosis of

IBD can interfere with the physical energy a child needs to do well in school and follow other pursuits, which can negatively affect a child's self-esteem. With the diagnosis of IBD, the apparent loss of control (for example, rectal bleeding, bowel movement accidents, and invasive procedures) challenges the child's need for mastery and skill development. This apparent loss of control can cause anxiety and feelings of helplessness. Children may also be fearful about falling behind in school, and their fear or actual lagging behind might make them feel isolated from others their age.

Children may choose not to perform certain activities that might show that they are "different" because of their IBD. Feeding tubes or central venous catheters (devices for easy vein access) can be a big source of insecurity for children. At a time when children are having their first sleepovers, even taking medication in front of friends can be embarrassing. Not being able to go to school because the disease is active can distance children from friends. They may feel overwhelmed and unable to catch up when they are ready to return.

Children of this age still use real-world concrete thinking, and they may also still have unusual beliefs about why they are sick or why they need to go to the hospital (for example, they may perceive going to the hospital or having medical tests as punishment). As they mature, they begin to understand difficult information about how the gastrointestinal system works, though they may still have mistaken ideas about what causes problems. A child may understand that he is having abdominal pain because the IBD is irritating his intestines but may still secretly believe it is because of an unrelated event, such as being unkind to his sibling. Discuss these feelings with your child. Understanding your child's worries can help you encourage him to overcome them. Finding and encouraging his strengths can improve self-esteem.

School-age children may become more and more focused on the effects of the treatments on their bodies and may begin to display fears of bodily harm and death. Middle-school-age children tend to focus on the present. Because of this, it is best to tell them about procedures no more than one week ahead. This will help them handle the situation best and decrease the possibility of intense negative reactions.

Ask your child questions to make sure he understands the facts about IBD and its treatment. Let your child know it is acceptable to have negative feelings about the diagnosis, such as fear, frustration, and anger. Many children in this age group will express their feelings, ideas, and fantasies about IBD through play, such as drawing or role-play—they may play doctor, for example. Encourage your child's use of these methods to help him cope with IBD-related stresses, such as medication, IVs, or injections. Use techniques such as distraction and relaxation to help him express his feelings during procedures.

Educating your child's friends and their parents about your child's IBD can help create a supportive environment. Excusing your child from the normal responsibilities that his peers and siblings have (homework, picking up, clearing the table, and other chores) can send a harmful message. It can make the child's fear and worry worse, or the child might begin to use symptoms to avoid doing unpleasant tasks. Your expectations of your child need to be reasonable, taking into account your child's health. If you have questions about appropriate expectations, talk with your child's pediatrician, pediatric gastroenterologist, or a psychologist.

IBD can present challenges that are too difficult for families to face alone. In these instances, outside help is a key to success. Making regular visits to your child's pediatrician or pediatric gastroenterologist will help make sure that the disease is under control and that your child is growing well. Other specialists may become important members of your child's health care team, too:

- Dieticians or nutritionists can help with your child's nutrition and, as a result, their growth.
- Psychologists can help children and families cope with the emotional challenges of IBD.
- Child-life specialists can help the family prepare for stressful procedures and cope with hospitalizations.
- Physical and occupational therapists can help your child get back to her best possible activity level after a period of serious illness.

- The school nurse and your child's teachers can help ensure the best educational environment for your child; talk with them about your child's IBD so that they understand your family's needs.

Your child's pediatrician or pediatric gastroenterologist can help you identify and contact these specialists.

Adolescence: Ages 13 through 17

Adolescence (the teen years) is the exciting transition from childhood to adulthood, beginning with puberty in early adolescence (12 to 14 years old) and ending with late adolescence (17 to 19 years old). This is a time of physical, emotional, and cognitive maturation, often with maturation in these different areas developing at different rates.

Adolescents begin to move from concrete thinking (thinking in terms of what is real or what exists) to abstract thought (having theories about the world around them). Adolescents tend to think more about their actions and the reasons they act in a certain way. The teenager's main task is to develop a sense of self-identity in order to move successfully from the family world to the outside adult world. Teenagers are very concerned with being accepted by their friends—their friends' approval is often more important to teens than their family's approval.

The rapid physical changes associated with puberty produce sharp self-awareness as well as concern about appearance. Poor growth or delayed sexual maturation, which many teens with IBD have compared with their healthy peers, can make concerns about appearance worse. Medical procedures that involve loss of function can be particularly difficult (a colostomy, for example). Accepting authority and giving up control to their medical team can lead teens to feel helpless and dependent. These are particularly difficult feelings in this age group. For all these reasons, adolescents with IBD may become challenging or rebellious when it comes to medical treatments, in an effort to regain a sense of control.

Teens have a growing understanding of the complicated causes of IBD, both environmental and genetic. This new awareness may increase fears about the possible long-term effects of IBD and its treatments. At this stage, concerns about what the disease might mean for the rest of the teen's life increase. Teens with chronic illnesses are likely to overstate the possible restrictions that come with their condition (for instance, "I'll never be able to play sports"). Or they may choose to participate in risky behavior (such as smoking) to be accepted by their friends.

Most people with IBD believe that stress can make the symptoms of their disease worse, and accumulating medical evidence shows that they are right. There is no doubt that IBD causes stress for teens, their parents, and their siblings. Even without symptoms of active disease, the teenager often worries about whether the symptoms will come back and prevent him from going on a school field trip, being on the basketball team, or going to the senior prom.

The stress is greater when teens have symptoms of active disease. They worry about making multiple trips to the bathroom while trying to attend school, or about how the medicine they take will change the way they look. An even bigger stress occurs during the complete disruption of their life due to surgery or a stay in the hospital.

Parents are often stressed by the competing demands of a career and caring for an ill child. Siblings are also affected. They are concerned about their brother or sister's health, and they often feel left out. They feel that they are not always told what is happening and that talks affecting their lives take place without them (see chapter 15).

When a teenager's lifestyle and activities are affected by the symptoms of IBD, or by worry and depression related to the disease, the problem must be recognized. Such reactions are normal and appropriate, and your teen needs support. Support groups are often helpful for adults with IBD, but less so for teenagers. If they feel well and have no symptoms, teens would rather think the disease does not exist, ignore it, and not talk about it. If they have symptoms that they cannot ignore (though they may try), they often do not want their friends to know about it, and they do not want to talk about it with their peers.

More than most chronic diseases, IBD can have a very strong effect on the life of a teen. With encouragement, trust, and respect for privacy, teenagers will express their anger and frustration about their disease. They can do so with adult family members, an adult friend, or their doctor. When they do talk about it, they should be shown ways to cope and to minimize the interruption in their life. Sometimes learning coping skills from a professional counselor is helpful.

The teen years are an important developmental period, when young people learn to adjust their emotions in ways that work best in different situations. Although mood swings can be normal, teens diagnosed with IBD appear to be at risk for developing serious depression. Parents must watch for early warning signs of depression:

- constant sadness or irritability
- changes in sleep habits
- loss of interest in fun activities
- withdrawal from friends and family

Report these symptoms to your child's doctor so that evaluation and treatment of the depression can start as early as possible.

For the teen who is trying hard to develop independence, maintain privacy, and gain acceptance from his peers, IBD is an embarrassing and, at times, humiliating disease. It can be especially difficult for a teen to discuss bowel habits and to tolerate invasive physical exams and tests. Thus, an open and trusting relationship between the teenager and his doctor is essential. Teenagers deserve to know that their doctor will tell them the truth about their disease and not hold back information. They should be able to trust that their doctor will answer questions completely and honestly. Furthermore, in most situations, the doctor's physical exam and conversation with the teenager should be done privately. Separate time should be set aside for discussion with the teenager, the parents, and the doctor together. The teen should always be part of discussions regarding major changes in the treatment plan.

Older teenagers insist on more independence and begin thinking about life after high school, including living away from home. They should slowly be given more responsibility for their own health. One example of increased responsibility is letting teens be in charge of taking their medicines, while ensuring that parents keep a check on the adherence by helping with refilling prescriptions. If teens are refilling their own prescriptions, parents should check to make sure prescriptions are refilled on time.

Doctors can also give older teenagers direct access to them, by offering them their business card with contact information. Although many teenagers do not use it, they do carry the card or keep it at home. The card is a powerful reminder of their independence, and of their doctor's trust in them.

The severity of IBD is not always related to the severity of the disease's effect on a teenager's life. Both parts—the severity of the disease and effects of the disease—must be recognized and addressed by everyone involved in the teen's life. By promoting independence, you can help your teen develop self-confidence and a sense of being able to take care of herself, even in the face of a chronic, challenging illness like IBD. In this way, teens with IBD can reach their full potential as adults.

Late Adolescence and Young Adulthood: Ages 18 through 21

All young adults face a challenge when they begin to consider what they will do after high school, be it going to college, getting a job, or moving away from home. Many consider distance from home and family to be a major part of their decision. Young adults with IBD also face the challenge of leaving behind health care providers and family members who have been their support system while living with IBD.

Young adults need to know that their goals and hopes for the future come first. For example, a young person may want very much to attend a university that is clear across the country from where she has been receiving medical care, because the school offers exactly what she is looking for. She should be encouraged to attend that school regardless of her IBD. Her physician should make every effort to identify a doctor who cares for IBD patients at her college's location. If a young person has no interest in going to college or leaving home, IBD should not be used as an excuse in making that decision.

Fortunately, young adults have more mature coping skills than children do, and they are able to handle the consequences of IBD better, but naturally they feel apprehensive about how IBD might affect their ability to perform at school or at work. If they experience health-related problems at school or at work, they deserve support and encouragement. They may also want to consider modifying their schedule. A few careers might not be possible for someone with IBD (as is true with any other chronic disease), but luckily those careers are few.

Many teenagers and young adults believe that IBD interferes with dating. Young adults start to wonder how IBD may affect their long-term relationships and their chances of becoming parents. They may worry about this issue even though they do not intend to start a family in the near future. Their doctor or mental health professional can give them reassuring information.

IBD undoubtedly interferes with the lives of people of all ages, and it affects their family and friends as well. For some, IBD can be easy to ignore. For others, it is a major inconvenience and can be a disabling disease. Nevertheless, IBD should not and need not prevent anyone from setting and achieving goals in sports, leisure activities, education, career, and family. Children, teens, and young adults are able to cope better and have more reasonable expectations when they are given encouragement, support, and accurate information.

Parents and caregivers play a critical role in helping their child cope with, and accept, an IBD diagnosis as easily as possible. The following guidelines can be helpful for parents and caregivers of children of all ages:

- Be open and honest, and use language your child understands when discussing the diagnosis of IBD with her.
- Help your child understand that showing feelings is normal and is a part of the learning experience in dealing with a chronic illness.
- Observe your child for constantly extreme emotional or behavioral reactions; if such reactions are present, consider getting

support for your child in the form of counseling or support groups.

- View your child as having IBD. Do not let IBD define your child. Observing this distinction will help you support your child's healthy move to adulthood.

回 17

Following the Treatment Plan

Adherence (also called *compliance*) means following the doctor's advice and recommended treatment. It means always taking the medications the doctor prescribed, following the recommended diet, and making any other necessary changes in lifestyle, as recommended by the doctor or other specialist. Adherence is a major concern for professionals who care for patients with chronic illnesses such as IBD.

Studies have shown that when a doctor recommends a plan or prescribes a medication to a patient with a chronic illness, the patient complies only about half the time. There are two main reasons for nonadherence with medical recommendations. The first is that the patient or the family does not agree with the doctor's plan, and the second is that the patient feels worse when he starts taking the medication, so he stops taking it. When the patient or his family members do not share their concern with the doctor, or the doctor doesn't explain the potential side effects of the treatment, problems with adherence can occur.

Young children will need their parents' help in adhering to medical treatment. For parents and older children, adherence is easier when they understand *why* they are having a problem adhering to medical advice. If the issues are clear, then the patient, family, and doctor can address the issues together.

If you or your child are not following the recommendations of your child's doctor, consider whether any of the following issues apply:

- Do you and your child understand IBD, including the fact that the disease is long lasting and requires long-term treatment? Do you understand the complications that can occur if the disease is left untreated, or if it does not respond to treatment?
- Has your doctor told you and your child what side effects to expect from the treatment (whether the treatment is medication, diet, or something else)?
- Does good communication and trust exist between you, your child, your family, and your health care provider?
- Are family or social influences causing problems with adherence? One example is a family in which the parents are separated, and the child with IBD spends time in two households.
- Have family members had past experience with health care providers that affects their acceptance of prescribed treatments? Or does the family have cultural beliefs that affect acceptance of prescribed treatments?
- Is your child concerned about the stigma of being seen taking medications? Or does she have concerns about other visible signs of having the disease (for example, feeding tubes)?
- Is your child's stage of development interfering with compliance? The age of a person with IBD can affect adherence; teenagers especially, as part of their normal development, may rebel against authority.
- Is the treatment plan complicated? A complicated treatment plan—medication schedule, difficult-to-follow diet—may cause problems with adherence.

What Can You Do to Ensure Adherence to the Medical Plan?

Your child needs to get the greatest benefit from her medications and other treatments. The following section offers guidelines to make sure your child and the rest of the family receive all the benefits of the medical advice provided to them.

Education

- You and your child (if she is old enough) should understand her medications. Your doctor can give you information about what the medications should do, and what possible side effects they have. When you get the prescription filled, your pharmacist can give you more information.
- If you are worried about the side effects of the medications, talk about your concerns with your child's doctor and the IBD team.
- Some side effects are routine, expected, and predictable, while others may be a concern, so you need to have a good understanding of the potential side effects. Some medications have side effects when your child first starts taking them, but the side effects may get better as your child's body gets used to the medication.

Treatment

- Work with your child's doctor to come up with a treatment plan that your child can adhere to.
- If not being able to sleep is one of the side effects of the medicine, your child may be able to take the medicine in the morning. If being sleepy is a side effect, your child could take the medicine at night. Check with your child's doctor or pharmacist to make sure it is okay to take the medicines at these different times.
- It is important to take the medications at regular times every day. They work best if the amount of medicine in the blood is always the same.
- If you or your child are tempted to stop any of his medication, think hard about it first. Some medications take several months before they start to work. If your child stops taking them, it may be several more months before they can start working again. Your child could get sick during that time, without medication to keep

his symptoms under control. Do not stop a medication without first talking to your child's doctor.

- Many medicines keep the symptoms of IBD from returning. If giving medications to your child when he feels well seems to make no sense to you, remember how your child felt when the disease was active.
- If you have trouble remembering when to give your child medicine, try a few tricks:

  Give him his pills at the same time every day.

  Link giving the pills with another activity that your child does at the same time every day, like taking a shower or brushing his teeth.

  Put sticky notes in a place where you will see them, like on a mirror. Change the place of the notes occasionally so that you do not get used to seeing them and start ignoring them.

  Use a weekly medication dispenser (available at your pharmacy) to help keep track of whether doses of medication were taken or not.

  Set up reminders on a smartphone.

- Store the medications properly, in sealed original containers with the label intact, and in a cool, dry place—unless the medication should be kept in the refrigerator.
- Renew the prescription before it runs out. Don't leave it to the last minute. If your child is a teenager, and it is his responsibility to renew the prescription, you should still have an understanding that he will let you know when the medication runs low.
- Remember to get new prescriptions written at the regular doctor's appointment to avoid delays that might cause the medicine to run out.

If your child is still having trouble taking his medications, try to figure out why.

- Maybe taking them is a "hassle."
- Maybe she just wishes IBD would go away.

- Maybe he has a difficult medication schedule.
- Maybe she doesn't like the side effects.

With good communication between patients, families, and health care providers, many of the problems of adherence can be solved. Find out what your child's concerns are and make sure the doctor knows about them, too. Ask your child's doctor to help you and your family come up with a plan for handling these concerns.

Self-Management Support

Self-management means taking responsibility for one's own well-being, behavior, and health. For this to happen, patients and families must be provided with the tools, skills, and support they need to improve their own well-being. For self-management in dealing with chronic illness to be successful, patients and their families need to:

- Understand their central role in managing the illness
- Make informed decisions about care
- Engage in healthy behaviors

Several organizations (see chapter 22) have online resources that can provide education and guidance about how to improve self-management, prepare for clinic visits, and communicate with your child's health care team.

▣ 18

School Days

Going to school to get a good education is an important task of childhood. School is also where much of a child's social and emotional growth occurs. Therefore, with some exceptions, the ability to attend school regularly is an important measure of good health. School provides an education in the whole experience of new expectations, learning to live with schedules, and dealing with teachers, friends, and new challenges. School is also about boyfriends and girlfriends, clubs, lunch hour, the gym, and a lot more.

Children with any chronic disease are at some risk for failing at school. Like all kids, children with inflammatory bowel disease find the school experience at times stimulating, boring, scary, and confusing. The emotional highway between the brain and the bowel is never busier than when a child is at school. Even healthy children experience stress from academic and social expectations—stress that can result in symptoms such as nausea, abdominal pain, and diarrhea. Since the connection between the gut and the brain is so strong, it is not surprising that some children with IBD experience uncomfortable symptoms while at school.

When a child is sick, the school experience may be exhausting and overwhelming. As with any chronic disease, however, normal activity is good medicine. Getting to school and seeing friends is a good distraction from symptoms. Keeping busy helps a child work up an appetite and makes her tired enough to fall asleep at night. This daily rhythm is important to the development of a healthy body and just as important to the medical care of the illness.

Although a child or teenager with IBD may not be able to make it through a full day of school on some occasions, it is still important for her to participate in school activities. Doing so may require some negotiations with teachers or the school principal. We advise parents to reserve home schooling for the worst times of illness, such as during recovery from surgery.

Discuss frequent school absences with the medical team. If your child is missing a lot of school, he may need better medications or counseling, or both.

Better medicine sometimes means stronger medicine. Many people with IBD try to minimize the amount, strength, or number of medicines they take. They feel that taking medicine is a sign of weakness, or that it is not "natural." Most doctors agree that you should take as few medicines as possible when you are well. If you have a medical condition, however, you are better off taking a medication that helps you lead a more normal life, even if the thought of taking medication is worrisome or scary.

If your child has to take medication at school, you can talk to his teachers about the best way to store the medicine and how your child can take it with the least disruption to his regular school schedule. Alternatively, your child's IBD doctor or the clinic nurse can make suggestions about how to fit the medication schedule into the school schedule.

Your child's IBD doctor can also help with planning for school trips outside your area. The doctor can create a medication plan that will minimize the chances of a flare, but it is still a good idea to have an emergency action plan just in case. This emergency plan should include a list of medications to treat a flare and, if possible, the name of a local medical contact, in case problems occur.

There are a few special challenges for kids with IBD at school. For one thing, everyone hates being embarrassed. Some kids are embarrassed because having IBD and taking medication makes them feel different. Others are humiliated if they must request many trips to the bathroom. Sharing the diagnosis with a few close friends is probably the best medicine for this problem. Also, the teacher may agree to allow the child to leave the room unobtrusively if he needs to go to the bathroom.

Most kids find that close friends will come together around them. The child or teen might practice talking to friends beforehand through role-play with his family or counselor. This gives him a chance to find the words he is comfortable using with his friends.

The expectations at school can sometimes become a problem. Teachers are used to hearing excuses all day long. Children in a wheelchair do not have to "make excuses" and explain that they have problems walking, but children with an "invisible" illness like IBD sometimes do not get the same consideration. This is where communication becomes so important. Most teachers will try to be helpful if they know the whole story. You or your child's doctor can provide teachers with information. That information can help your child and her teachers set reasonable expectations regarding schoolwork, assignment deadlines, and tests. It can also help to ask for unrestricted bathroom privileges in advance.

You can also set up a Section 504 plan in conjunction with the school administration. The "504" refers to the section of the federal Rehabilitation Act that ensures accommodations for children with disabilities. Templates for 504 plans are available on the Internet (see chapter 22) and include accommodations like bathroom privileges, medication administration by the school nurse, increased time between classes, seat assignments in class, and timed stop-the-clock testing. For older adolescents heading to college, contacting the college ahead of time would be a good way to ensure that these kinds of accommodations are put in place before your child shows up on the first day of classes. The school may also adjust your child's class schedule as well as housing with shared rooms or bathrooms.

Your child may experience particular problems dealing with the bathrooms at school. School bathrooms are rarely supervised, and they can be scary places. It is important that you, a counselor, or the teachers help your child or teenager solve these problems. Solutions include using the school nurse bathroom and carrying a deodorizer spray.

Without a doubt, other issues will come up at school. Many IBD programs have support groups that meet face-to-face or on the Internet. You may find that your child with IBD has a lot in common with children who have different illnesses. The ability to problem solve with other children of the same age can help your child find solutions that make her feel more comfortable at school and at home. The process of helping someone else with her problems is one of the more effective ways for a child with a chronic condition to adjust to her own condition and grow stronger.

Growing up involves taking chances, but it is mostly about learning to make good choices. School offers children, especially those with a chronic illness, many opportunities to make hard choices and learn from them. Some studies found that kids with IBD are stronger, more mature, and have better self-esteem than kids without serious diseases. Repeatedly making hard choices is like physical conditioning. "Reps" make the child or teen stronger.

回 19

Insurance and Other Financial Issues

Both Crohn's disease and ulcerative colitis are conditions that require long-term medical follow-up and treatment. The costs of care greatly vary depending on the disease severity. Patients with mild disease may have affordable medical expenses, but those with severe disease will experience considerable expense. Many of the new medications are very expensive; for example, one year of infliximab infusions can cost more than twenty thousand dollars. Hospitalizations lead to additional costs as well. For these reasons, it is essential to have health insurance and the associated peace of mind.

In the United States, employers provide many different types of health insurance policies. The policies vary significantly, with some providing only catastrophic coverage (going into effect only for a prolonged hospitalization), and others providing comprehensive outpatient and inpatient coverage. In general, if a family has a child with IBD, the family should, if at all possible, obtain a comprehensive insurance policy with a low co-pay for outpatient visits and a generous drug benefit plan. This way, if the child requires an expensive medication, it is more likely to be covered by insurance.

Because of the expense of several newer medications (such as the anti-TNFα medications), many insurers review the medical plan after the physician prescribes the medication. A nurse reviewer or physician at the insurance company will ask the physician to fill out a form with pertinent aspects of the patient's history (this is called a prior authorization form). Based on the medical information the company receives, they will either approve or deny the physician's prescription. A denial is not always permanent; it often means that the insurance company requires additional information about the patient's medical condition before it considers paying for a very expensive drug. Such information may include the patient's diagnosis; what other therapies have been tried in the past; published medical evidence that the prescribed drug is effective; and alternative treatments to be considered. As a child with IBD becomes a young adult, he must also be aware of the need to keep health insurance. The types of health insurance plans offered by an employer may be one factor in determining where the young adult chooses to work (see chapter 19). With the enactment of the Affordable Care Act (ACA) in 2010, young adults in the United States could stay on their parents' health insurance until the age of 26. Many parents and their children who worried about losing health insurance after the children moved away from home or graduated from college no longer needed to worry. Future changes in health care law, however, could change this benefit.

Family and Medical Leave

Although most children with IBD are healthy and can participate in all school and extracurricular activities, at times the illness may require extra parental attention and involvement. This is particularly true in children with more severe forms of Crohn's disease or ulcerative colitis, or children undergoing surgery. In some cases, a parent may need to take time off from work to care for the ill child. In the United States, the Family Medical Leave Act (FMLA) allows employees to formally request *unpaid* leave from their employers for up to twelve weeks in a year to care for an immediate family member with a serious health condition. Requirements to be eligible for FMLA include working for the same employer for at least twelve months and working for a company that employs at least fifty people. Although FMLA does not provide pay for family members who choose to take time off from work, it does protect employees from being fired because they are caring for a sick relative. To apply for FMLA leave, both the employee (parent) and the child's physician must complete paperwork documenting the nature of the child's medical condition.

Disability Benefits

Most people with IBD lead healthy lives or have mild symptoms and are therefore not eligible for disability. Under rare circumstances, however, the IBD may be so severe that a child or young adult may be eligible for disability benefits (Supplemental Security Income, or SSI). Being approved for SSI may allow a child to be eligible for Medicaid benefits. Applying for SSI is a long and difficult process that usually requires the assistance of an attorney. Careful documentation of "marked and severe functional limitations that are expected to last at least 12 months" is required. Such limitations may include severe anemia, malabsorption, malnutrition, obstruction, or abdominal abscess.

The regulations regarding insurance coverage and patient's rights change rapidly, and it is possible that by the time this book is published, different federal or state regulations will be in place. What's important is that parents and children with IBD know that both federal and state regulations are in place to protect families coping with a chronic illness. Excellent resources for families who have questions relating to financial concerns, insurance coverage, and employee leave include social workers or financial advocates at hospitals and attorneys who specialize in disability and medical insurance. Some organizations provide resources on the Internet as well (see chapter 22).

Part V
As a Child Grows Up

▣ 20

Transitions from School to Work and Independent Living

Children growing up with a chronic illness such as inflammatory bowel disease face even more challenges than other children their age. This chapter highlights some of the more common physical and emotional problems faced by a child with IBD during some of life's normal transitions.

Transition to Middle School

Many physical and emotional changes and challenges accompany the transition from elementary school to middle school.

Physical Development and Puberty

As with other chronic conditions, IBD may cause a delay in puberty. Children with IBD may be smaller than all their friends. Girls may not start their periods or may have delayed breast development. These delays are not usually a cause for long-term concern. Children with IBD should be reassured that even if they enter puberty later than their friends do, they will eventually catch up. Like all children, those with IBD should be given information about the physical changes that will happen during puberty. Let your child know that these changes are part of the natural process of growing into adulthood.

A number of factors influence the timing of puberty (sexual maturation):

- family traits
- hormones—the chemicals in the body that cause puberty
- nutrition factors or weight issues
- disease activity and the location of your child's disease

Delays in puberty can be the result of malnutrition, not getting enough calories in the diet, or malabsorption (when our bodies cannot take in the vitamins and nutrients they need from the food we eat).

In girls, the first sign of puberty is usually breast budding, which starts on average at the age of 10 years, but it can happen as late as age 13. Menstruation (getting a period) usually starts about two years after the start of puberty. You should talk to your daughter's health care provider if she has no puberty-related changes by age 13, or if she does not get her period by age 15.

Boys normally enter puberty one year later than girls do. The first signs are enlargement of the testes and thinning and reddening of the scrotum (the sac containing the testes). These signs usually occur at age 11, but in boys with IBD, they may be delayed until age 14, or even later.

Steady growth during middle childhood results in height increases of about 2 inches per year in girls and boys. Weight increases on average by approximately 6 pounds per year. One of the first signs of IBD may be a short build, especially if the child has Crohn's disease. If the disease has been under good control for several months, and your child is not growing in height, you should talk with his doctor. The doctor might recommend testing for other disorders (for example, thyroid disease, celiac disease, or diabetes).

Nutrition

Good nutrition is very important for a young person's overall health and well-being (see chapter 13). A varied and balanced diet supports growth, energy, and general health. For best growth, your child should be eating a diet high in calories. The diet must also be rich in calcium to support bone growth and strength. A low-fiber, low-residue diet is recommended only if narrowing is present in the bowel (low-residue diets leave very little material in the bowel). Talking with a dietician about the best diet for your child's particular needs can be helpful.

While certain foods might make the symptoms of IBD worse in some people, there are no specific foods that your child should avoid. No evidence shows that inflammation of the intestines is affected by the food a person eats. Middle school, however, is a common time for lactose (milk sugar) intolerance to appear. Inability to break down the sugar in milk and other dairy products can lead to gas, bloating, abdominal pain, cramps, and diarrhea. An easy, noninvasive test known as a *lactose breath test* can diagnose this condition. An over-the-counter dietary supplement containing the enzyme *lactase*, which breaks down the milk sugar, is available to take with dairy products to prevent development of symptoms.

Coping with the Stress of Illness in Middle School

Children with IBD often have more stress in their daily lives than others their age do. For example, they must cope with taking medications once or multiple times per day, frequent doctor visits or hospitalizations, painful examinations, injections or blood draws, body-image issues related to delayed growth and puberty, and sometimes surgery. Although no one can avoid stress completely, the following suggestions may make things a little easier:

- Always inform your child of what lies ahead concerning medical tests and treatments. A child's worry is often due to fear of the unknown.
- Listen to your child and encourage him to express emotions, whether he is sad, frustrated, angry, or fearful. Be supportive and always try to listen to what he is *not* saying (in other words, try to read between the lines).
- Talk openly about the illness so your child feels comfortable with the topic.
- Talking to other children who have gone through the same or similar experiences can be valuable. Your child may relate well to other children with IBD. It often helps your child to realize that

he is not the only one with this condition. Other children with IBD (and perhaps their parents) may be able to share helpful coping strategies for home and school.

- Focus on your child's strengths and talents. A child with IBD often feels discouraged. Many children with IBD are also angry about the restrictions placed on physical activity, or about the discomfort of the disease. Many children derive great pleasure and pride from various creative activities, such as playing a musical instrument, drawing, painting, or writing. A hobby such as collecting coins, stamps, or baseball cards can also be fun and instill feelings of success. In addition, academic success should always be encouraged and rewarded. Like adults, all children need to feel a sense of accomplishment.

- Encourage your child to begin to take an active role in his health care (if he is not already doing so). Allow him to participate in the decision-making process whenever possible. For example, allow your child to pick which arm to use for a blood draw. Also, allow for some flexibility in scheduling an endoscopic procedure or x-rays so that your child can weigh in on the decision. If a bowel preparation is needed prior to the tests, give the middle school child some options. Options will help your child follow the bowel preparation procedures more willingly and give him a sense of control.

School Issues for the Child with Inflammatory Bowel Disease

During the middle school years, children want to look and behave as their peers do and participate in the same activities. They want acceptance from their classmates, possibly more than at any other time in their school years. They shape their self-esteem and self-image by this acceptance.

Keep teachers informed and updated regarding changes in your child's medical condition. For example, if your child's appearance has changed, meet with your child's teachers before she returns to school. Teacher meetings are the key to preventing unnecessary problems in your child's progress at school. Children spend most of their time in school, and teachers may be the first to notice a flare of the disease. They can let you know about changes in behavior, lack of attention, and signs of depression or anxiety. Teachers can also tell you how your child interacts with classmates, and they will keep you updated on academic performance.

Relationships with Peers

IBD can present a special challenge for children as they relate to their age group. Any condition that requires medications, individual bathroom privileges, or frequent absences from school can result in embarrassment. When helped by their friends, family, teachers, and health care professionals, children can develop into stronger individuals, overcoming many barriers.

Some parents urge their children to hide their illness and medications from peers, fearing that their children might have to endure ridicule if others are aware of the condition. This may send a wrong message to the child, telling her that IBD is a shameful condition, needing concealment. Instead, children should be encouraged to disclose the condition to close contacts in a comfortable setting. Telling close friends can greatly ease the isolation many children with IBD feel. A teacher or the school nurse may be helpful in guiding children through the process of telling their friends about their illness.

Sports

Children with IBD should participate in sports if they want to. Studies show that bones become stronger and denser when physical activity is increased. Children with IBD should avoid spending too much free time watching TV or playing video games. These inactive hobbies may actually damage bone growth and add to decreased bone density (resulting in weaker bones). Coaches, parents, teachers, and health care providers should be supportive of a child's athletic activities. In return, the child with IBD should do his part by taking prescribed medications, eating a balanced diet, drinking plenty of fluids, and getting plenty of rest.

Transition to College Away from Home

Many young people with IBD find the adjustment to college to be more complex than they expected because of health issues they need to deal with. Being away at college is often the first time in a young adult's life that she is managing her own health without a parent's daily assistance. There are new routines, and sometimes no routines. Finding the college that is the best fit is a challenge for everyone, so a student with IBD needs to realize that her illness should be only one among many factors she needs to consider while choosing a college. A young adult with IBD is more than a patient, and if she is unhappy with her choice of school, health and studies are likely to suffer.

IBD should not preclude exploring academic institutions away from home. The decision to attend college far from home or as a commuting student is an individual one. Still students with IBD should anticipate some considerations to help make their transition to college as seamless as possible while they maintain the continuity of their health care.

Preparations

As soon as a college or university has been selected and the student has been accepted, contact the school's Office of Disability Services or Dean of Students Office. This helps establish with the school that it might need to make accommodations for the student with IBD so that if the student needs to make future or unpredictable requests, he has less work to do in the moment of medical need. This is also the office to use for residential accommodations, including requests for

- a private bathroom
- a private room
- permission for a refrigerator in the dorm room
- permission for a car on campus (if appropriate)

Many students with IBD had Section 504 plans in high school that provided academic accommodations so that their studies were not compromised. Section 504 plans are written agreements between parents and schools that provide reasonable accommodations for children with disabilities. For a child with IBD, a 504 plan may also outline a disease management plan. College authorities can often help the student develop similar plans to provide accommodations in scheduling or housing in the college environment. Revising the high school 504 plan so that it is relevant to the particular school's curriculum is usually done through the Disabilities Office or the Dean of Students, and this should be initiated as soon as possible.

Before the student heads off to college, he should find out what services are provided by the university health clinic, such as labs, pharmacies, and radiology services. For the student on maintenance medications, it is helpful to scout out where prescriptions can be filled when on campus. Many families have drug plans that provide Internet access to pharmacies that directly ship medications to students living out of town. If this service is not available, traveling to college with at least a month's supply of daily medications is a good idea because it allows time to set up with a new pharmacy and have prescriptions transferred to be filled locally.

For students not attending school close to home, plans should be made to identify a gastroenterologist near the school campus. Students may still see their primary gastroenterologist at scheduled visits or may decide it is time to transfer care. Either way, it is important to have a physician close by in the event of sudden illness. An initial appointment should be scheduled as soon as possible after arriving on campus so that the new gastroenterologist can review the student's complete history, medication schedule, and test results.

Lifestyle Considerations

Once on campus, the new student with IBD will have much to consider. Many people with IBD have certain foods in their diet that cause symptoms or flares. Parents need to be realistic about their child's college eating habits; there will always be leftover dinner for breakfast and vice versa. It is the student's responsibility to make attempts to eat correctly and to maintain a nutritious diet.

Often, the dietician at the campus dining halls can provide guidance on menus at the various campus or dorm locations as well as options that can easily be made available as standing alternatives to meal plans. Students receiving nutritional supplements may want to identify a primary dining hall for use and ask the disability support services to keep some supplements in the cafeteria refrigerator for easy access without the student having to return to the dorm.

College can also demand the development of new strategies and creative ways for the student with IBD to maintain a healthy lifestyle. Once on campus, it may be helpful to make note of the locations of campus bathroom facilities, both inside and outside academic buildings, as well as the hours they remain open. Remembering to take medications can be more difficult with new schedules and many more distractions. In this high-tech age, reminders can come in many forms: cell phone alarms, watch alarms, pop-up reminders on a laptop or wireless technology; low-tech also works—sticky notes or taping medicine bottles to the mirror.

College campuses provide many opportunities for students to engage in risk-taking behavior. Such behavior is an even bigger gamble for students with chronic illness than it is for other students. Exposure to and use of alcohol and recreational drugs are dangerous in general but can be especially harmful to students with IBD. Students with IBD not only face all the common risks, but also must consider how these substances interact with their prescribed medications and the risk of triggering a flare.

Disclosure: Who Should I Tell?

A common concern of students with IBD heading off to college is determining who to talk to about their condition. Staff of the student health service should always know about a student's medical history. Whether others should know, however, is a personal and private issue.

The student does not have to tell anybody about his diagnosis of IBD, but finding and sharing the diagnosis with someone trustworthy, who can provide support if a medical complication presents itself, especially if the student is away from home, is an important consideration. Many students decide to seek out, confide in, and rely on other students with IBD or another chronic medical condition.

The decision about how much to share, and with whom, should be guided by personal priorities and comfort level. Many students initially choose to tell only their roommates, and eventually they may share the diagnosis with close friends. Often, it is helpful to alert academic advisers or academic mentors, especially if questions arise about lighter schedules or curriculum selections.

The student at first may not know anyone who has medical issues such as IBD. Universities draw a wide array of students, however, and many students have medical issues they must contend with in addition to their academic studies. The college environment is now more accepting of the needs of students and even values the diversity that differences bring.

Checklist

In an effort to ease the transition to college and reduce additional stress amid an already significant life change, we created the following quick reference list of what your student should consider as she leaves home for college:

Medical Care

- Do I have all the vaccinations I need? Are they up to date?
- Who should I contact if I am not feeling well?
- How should I contact these identified individuals: by phone, by e-mail, via parents?
- What are the important phone numbers and e-mail addresses to take to school to allow easy contact with family members or physicians?
- How can medical team members best return my calls? What is the best route for the medical team to contact me: by voicemail, e-mail, pager, phone, my parents?
- What health services are available on campus?
- Has a local gastroenterologist near campus been identified?
- How can I schedule an introductory appointment in advance of a necessary appointment?

- Have copies of medical records been sent to the local doctor and university health services in advance?
- Where can I get blood draws and laboratory tests done?
- What is the fax number of the local laboratory?
- To whom and to what fax number or address should a local lab send test results?

Medications

- How much of an initial supply of medications should I bring to campus?
- Where can I store medications?
- Should I inform my roommate(s) of my medication schedule and medical needs? How will I explain this?
- What are the steps to take to avoid running out of medications, and what can I do if this still occurs?
- What is the local pharmacy's address? What are its phone and fax numbers?
- What are the requirements for sending prescriptions in advance to my new pharmacy?
- What is the most convenient and accessible avenue to keep medications refilled: local pharmacy or mail-order pharmacy?

Diet

- Can I tolerate the dining hall food?
- Will I have regular access to sufficient and adequate calories?
- Should I bring supplements to campus?
- Are there relevant food restrictions? Are there foods I cannot eat?
- How does alcohol interact with my IBD medication(s)?

Housing

- What will be the setting: dormitory, apartment, house?
- Will I have roommates?
- How accessible and private are the residential toilets?
- Where are the bathrooms located around campus?

Transitioning to college is exciting and scary at the same time, for student and for parents. There are many responsibilities, and even more possibilities, for the young adult heading to college. The healthier your child is, the more she can enjoy this exciting time and take advantage of all the opportunities that college can provide.

Transition to Work

Health Insurance Considerations

One of the most important issues that young adults with IBD must handle as they enter the workforce is maintaining health insurance coverage. Young adults who are full-time students can often stay on their parents' policy until age 26 under the Affordable Care Act. When a young adult is no longer a student, however, or reaches the maximum age covered by the policy, he can no longer be covered under his parents' insurance.

As health insurance is no longer an automatic benefit of employment in many circumstances, the employee must pay close attention to the benefits offered by his new employer. Because transitioning from school to the workforce usually involves the simultaneous transfer of health coverage from the family's plan to an employer's policy, the newly employed person with IBD must explore his employer's different health insurance policies. It is also necessary to compare the various coverage choices that may be offered by a single employer, including HMOs, PPOs, point of service (POS) plans, or fee-for-service plans.

When combing through the plans' options, consider

- frequency of visits covered
- number of visits covered within a calendar year
- flexibility and ability to choose specialists not only for IBD but also for associated problems, such as arthritis (rheumatologists), nutrition (dieticians), and coping (mental health professionals)

Take care to examine the fees associated with maintenance outpatient visits, emergency room visits, lab work, x-rays, inpatient hospital stays, and mental health coverage. The fees for these services should be balanced against the employee's cost of the plan and the flexibility the plan offers in choosing preferred providers. Though an HMO may be more affordable, the time spent obtaining referrals from a primary care physician for various subspecialty providers is often not worth the physical cost of prolonging access to necessary care, especially when such care will be a recurrent need.

Various health spending strategies are available through employers to help offset some of the high cost of health care:

- Health savings accounts (HSAs) are savings accounts that may receive contributions from an eligible individual or any other person, including an employer or a family member, on behalf of the eligible individual. Contributions, other than employer contributions, are deductible on the eligible individual's tax return. Employer contributions are not included in income. Distributions from an HSA that are used to pay qualified medical expenses are not taxed.

- Health flexible spending arrangements (FSAs) may receive contributions from an eligible individual. Employers may also contribute. Contributions are not included in income. Reimbursements from an FSA that are used to pay qualified medical expenses are not taxed.

- Health reimbursement arrangements (HRAs) must receive contributions from the employer only. Employees may not contribute. Contributions are not included in income. Reimbursements from an HRA that are used to pay qualified medical expenses are not taxed.

Because IBD is a chronic illness, one of the most critical considerations when transferring from a previous policy to a new employer's policy is that typically not more than sixty days elapse without coverage before the new policy becomes effective. If an employee has a gap in health insurance coverage for more than sixty days, the new policy has the right to decline coverage of any routine, maintenance, or emergency care related to a preexisting condition—such as IBD. If there is less than a sixty-day gap before the new policy takes effect, the new policy must cover the costs associated with any preexisting condition, including IBD.

The sixty-day rule is noteworthy because many employers' policies do not become effective immediately upon employment. Therefore, the employee must take care to make sure there is no gap between the termination of an old policy and the commencement of a new one. Often, a young person entering the workforce must purchase additional months on a parent's health plan through COBRA (the Consolidated Omnibus Budget Reconciliation Act), or have a discussion with a potential employer's human resources director about appealing the standard date of effective coverage through a company's plan.

Many young adults with IBD simply choose not to consider interviewing at agencies or companies that do not offer health insurance. People living with IBD have the benefit of *knowing* they have a chronic illness that can force unpredictable demands on their lives. Using that information to make an informed decision empowers the job seeker to be proactive in identifying options for reasonable coverage. If an ideal job opportunity does not offer adequate health insurance, a person has the option of purchasing private policies through major insurance carriers. These can be costly, but they are often less costly than a large hospital bill or the physical cost of not getting adequate maintenance care and suffering a potentially preventable flare.

Disclosure to Employer and Co-workers

A new or potential employee has no legal obligation to disclose any personal or health-related information to her employer if her condition does not substantially interfere with work responsibilities or performance. It is not necessary to tell a prospective employer about an IBD diagnosis during an interview. The interview is an occasion for an employer to assess a candidate's fit for the position based on skills. It is a time for a candidate to learn about the position, its associated responsibilities, and the resources and benefits available on the job so that she can determine if it fits her needs and goals.

Once the employee starts a new job, she faces new personal and professional challenges. One such personal challenge is deciding with whom and when to share personal facts. Outside the performance of work, all other aspects of one's life are personal, and personal information is shared with co-workers at the discretion of the employee. When a person has a condition such as IBD, however, it is necessary to consider how to best manage medical and employment responsibilities. If the symptoms of IBD act up, who among one's colleagues would be most affected? How might supervisors react? Would they be more understanding if they had the knowledge that IBD symptoms were affecting an employee's ability to work, or would they use the knowledge maliciously?

It is important to identify people who can be trusted, and then share the diagnosis when the time seems right. In many circumstances, telling an immediate supervisor before the employee necessarily feels comfortable telling peers or co-workers may be appropriate. Should IBD symptoms flare, or an unpredictable and urgent complication arise, it may be helpful if an immediate supervisor is aware that the employee has a condition that remits and relapses. Her understanding of the nature of IBD can minimize employment problems before they occur. It may, for example, prevent your employer from interpreting a last-minute absence from work soon after beginning a new job as reflecting a poor work ethic.

Assessing the Work Environment

With any potential job, make sure there is realistic and reasonable access to health care. While a person with IBD should not compromise his career goals, it is practical to consider the degree to which a particular job might make it difficult to obtain necessary health care in a timely manner. For example, a young adult patient with IBD had always looked forward to working on a cruise ship so that he could travel and see different parts of the country and world. This lifestyle clearly posed barriers to the continuity of health care. To reconcile this goal with the reality of knowing that his IBD required frequent attention, he applied only to major cruise lines with established health insurance plans, and he deliberately requested certain itineraries that docked at ports in major domestic and international cities. These cities had well-established medical centers.

IBD doesn't have to rule out jobs requiring work abroad. Most developed countries have physicians who can provide appropriate care if medical demands arise. Take the experience of another young adult patient who had always dreamed of doing missionary work. Rather than abandon this goal because of her IBD, she consulted with her gastroenterologist and selected assignments in areas of the world with developed medical centers that she could easily reach in case of emergency.

The physical environment of a job is also an important consideration, including accessibility to bathrooms. For instance, does a job opportunity require frequent travel? If so, by car or airplane? Would being on the road frequently lead to anxiety about access to bathrooms? Would it hinder optimal quality of life and success at work?

Reviewing environmental stressors and potential triggers of symptom flares is important when considering a new job. Some jobs may take place in a setting where there is a lot of cigarette smoking, something that might provoke an IBD attack. Working in a restaurant or bar, an employee might be more likely to eat the establishment's food, which in a person with IBD might encourage a diet that disagrees with his digestive system. In some industries and jobs, having a drink with a client is a large part of the culture, but such an activity might at times be difficult for someone with IBD. Therefore, being aware of what triggers your disease, how environmental factors stress your body, and the personal course of your IBD can influence your career choices. These factors do not necessarily mean you should not pursue or accept a particular job; however, for many individuals, these are practical issues to consider when IBD is part of daily life.

Choosing the Best Fit and Finding a New Routine

Ultimately, young adults should not design goals and career aspirations around their IBD. Yet, it is often necessary to reconcile the demands of IBD with career choices. How flexible is a workday? Does the company offer compensation time ("comp time," in which hours missed from work are made up at another time) for doctors' appointments, or does it require employees to use vacation or sick time for medical needs? If so, would this become a disincentive to taking the time to care for your health? If a person is out of work beyond a certain number of days, is she required to use short-term disability and receive lower pay?

Young adults with IBD need to rely on practical self-assessment and sensible self-monitoring, since it is often not clear how IBD might be affected by the demands of work. Work commitments can be even more erratic or demanding than those experienced in high school or college. As the job becomes familiar, it is often helpful to build in some sort of predictability so that the known demands of IBD can be incorporated into the workday. This can mean finding new times of day to take medications, or new places to keep a duplicate supply of medicine, so that a last-minute out-of-town meeting or the need to work exceptionally late for a deadline does not prevent access to maintenance medications. It can also mean packing a lunch or keeping select foods available in the office refrigerator to avoid dietary triggers. Reconciling issues such as these with your personal course of IBD will help you transition successfully into the workplace.

▣ 21

Transitions from Pediatric to Adult Health Care Providers

Most children with IBD in the United States receive their IBD-related medical care from pediatric gastroenterologists. When the children become young adults, however, they usually transition to an adult gastroenterologist. Such transitions are often challenging because the patient and the physician have become close over the years, and separation is difficult. In some countries, the transition from a pediatric to an adult GI practice is very sudden, occurring on schedule when a child turns a certain age. In the United States the transition often happens as young people are either entering or graduating college (or reaching college age) and is done when the patient and the pediatric physician mutually agree that the time for transition has arrived. Thus, the young adult has time both to mature and to prepare for the transition.

In addition to leaving a physician they are familiar with, young people transitioning from pediatric to adult GI practices may find they are leaving a *system* they are familiar with, too. The primary difference between a pediatric and an adult system is the health care provider's expectations of the patient. In a pediatrician's office, the parents attend every visit and often provide most of the patient history. For a child with a chronic illness, it is not uncommon for that pattern of parental input to persist in the pediatrician's office even after a child is mature and perfectly capable of doing most of her own talking. Once a child becomes a young adult and "graduates" to an adult practice, however, the parents may not even be allowed into the examining room. At this point, young people need to provide a complete history themselves, and take down all the doctor's recommendations and act on them without input from their parents. This may be a challenge for a young person who has been used to Mom and Dad taking care of things.

Taking Ownership of IBD While Becoming a Young Adult

The transition to the adult-based system is both inevitable and desirable; to help make the transition go smoothly, we recommend a graduated approach. This approach involves parents preparing the teenager starting in high school to acquire the skill set necessary to be both a "good patient" and an effective advocate for his own medical needs. As a parent, you can begin preparing your child in late middle school or high school for more independence and autonomy. Ask him to speak when he goes to the doctor, even if the doctor is looking at you. Over time, make sure your child knows what his diagnosis is (Crohn's disease or ulcerative colitis), where the disease is located (ileum, colon, etc.), and what medications and doses are prescribed. After your child is in middle to late high school, offer to step out of the room at an appropriate time, so your child and the doctor have some "alone time" together. This alone time serves two purposes: it enables the child to gain a sense of independence, and it allows the doctor to ask sensitive questions. During your child's later teenage years, the physician will be an important source of counseling about high-risk behaviors (sexual activity, smoking, alcohol) that should not be discussed in front of parents because it is important for the child to feel free to speak honestly and to ask the physician questions.

After your child turns 18, she is legally an adult and entitled to autonomy. At that point, you should discuss with her whether she wants you in the room during the visit. In addition, the doctor may ask your child for permission to disclose medical information to her parents. At this point, it is the patient, not the parents, who determines the degree of information sharing and involvement. Most patients, however, continue to rely on their parents as trusted advisers and welcome participation in the visits.

Once your child transitions to an adult practice, however, you will probably need to stay outside the exam room and learn about the details of the visit from your child.

In conclusion, the journey from childhood to adulthood is frightening for some individuals and exhilarating for others. Parents and physicians must support the transition to independence and empower the child to gain ever increasing amounts of responsibility. If a young adult is neglecting his health (for example, missing appointments, not taking medications, or not keeping health insurance), parents and providers need to encourage him to get back on track. At this vulnerable age, peer and patient support groups may be invaluable.

Part VI
Additional Helpful Information

🔲 22

Where to Get Additional Help and Information

If your child has just been diagnosed with inflammatory bowel disease, or has had the disease for a number of years but you have some new questions, where do you go for information? Ideally, at the time of diagnosis, you were given information on IBD. Some hospitals routinely provide newly diagnosed IBD patients with an information packet. Print brochures published by the Crohn's and Colitis Foundation are probably available in your gastroenterologist's office. If they are not, ask your physician to order some, or call your local Crohn's and Colitis Foundation chapter.

If you were not given any information, or if you have additional questions, the Internet is a quick and easy source. Typing "inflammatory bowel disease" into an Internet search engine will result in hundreds of thousands of pages you can visit. But there are problems and pitfalls in such searches. The first problem is the enormous amount of information you can find. The second is that these sites cannot be used as a reliable source of information when it comes to the care of *your* child. The information online is often based on general information, or on one person's experience. This experience may or may not be related to your child's IBD. So how do you begin to sort through this overwhelming amount of information? How do you know which information is right for you and your child?

Happily, there are several very good sources of information on the Internet. Even if you do not have Internet access at home, you can get access at school, at work, at your friends' houses, or at the public library.

This chapter is not meant to provide you with an exhaustive list of all available websites that provide information about IBD, but one of the first sites you should visit is that of the North American Society for Pediatric Gastroenterology, Hepatology and Nutrition, www.naspghan.org, which is a valuable resource for patients and parents of children with IBD. Among its other benefits, it allows parents to search for NASPGHAN-affiliated pediatric gastroenterologists (children's digestive disease specialists) in their area. From the NASPGHAN Web site, you can reach NASPGHAN'S parent and patient resource Web site by using the search term GI Kids, or you can go directly to www.gikids.org, to find additional information about IBD. Informational brochures on these sites can be found in several languages, including English, Spanish, French, and Portuguese.

Another early stop on the Internet should be the Crohn's and Colitis Foundation, at www.crohnsandcolitisfoundation.org. This is a comprehensive, reliable, and up-to-date information site about IBD in both children and adults. In addition to disease information, this site features webcasts on important topics, such as diet and nutrition tips for people with IBD, information on the latest research and clinical trials for IBD, and advice for how you can advocate for your child (for example, how to pursue a 504 plan for your child or request college accommodations). You can also find information about Crohn's and Colitis Foundation chapters in your area. If you join a chapter, you will receive newsletters and information on various activities, which may include support group sessions, IBD camps for kids, and fundraisers. The Crohn's and Colitis Foundation also sponsors a Web site that provides information about IBD geared toward adolescents (www.justlikemeibd.org).

A few other sites you may wish to visit include the National Institutes of Health (NIH), at www.nlm.nih.gov. On this site, if you search for "inflammatory bowel disease" you will find links to the latest news on CD and UC. The site also has a link to government-sponsored clinical trials, www.clinicaltrials.gov. The Centers for Disease Control and Prevention

(CDC), www.cdc.gov, and the American Gastroenterological Association, www.gastro.org, also have information about IBD. ImproveCare-Now, www.improvecarenow.org, is a collaborative community where patients, parents, and health care providers work together to improve the health of children with IBD. For information about complementary and alternative therapies, the National Institutes of Health's National Center for Complementary and Integrative Health (NCCIH), www.nccih.nih .gov, is a good starting place to search for up-to-date, unbiased information, including the "Herbs at a Glance" page.

Your library and local bookstore can be sources of good information, too. We recommend asking your doctors about appropriate books and educational materials if your child has IBD. Hospital patient libraries often have books and videos as well.

This is a busy time in the field of IBD. Information on causes and treatments is changing daily, so it is important to keep informed. The sources above will expand your knowledge of IBD. Remember, however, that no two people with IBD are alike. Individual help and advice is as close as your telephone—take advantage of your doctor's knowledge.

回 23

Frequently Asked Questions

What is inflammatory bowel disease?

Inflammatory bowel disease (IBD) is a general name for two different conditions: Crohn's disease (CD) and ulcerative colitis (UC). CD and UC cause damage to different parts of the digestive (gastrointestinal, or GI) tract and sometimes to other parts of the body as well.

What is Crohn's disease?

Crohn's disease is an ongoing disease that causes inflammation (swelling and irritation) of the digestive tract. Although it can involve any area of the GI tract from the mouth to the anus, it most commonly affects the small intestine, colon (large intestine), or both.

Why is my condition called Crohn's disease?

The disease is named after Dr. Burrill Crohn. In 1932, Dr. Crohn and two colleagues, Dr. Leon Ginzberg and Dr. Gordon Oppenheimer, published the first paper describing what is now known as Crohn's disease.

What is ulcerative colitis (UC)?

UC is a chronic disorder that causes inflammation (swelling and irritation) of the colon (large intestine).

How long have I had my IBD?

No one knows for sure. Some people can have symptoms for a long time, even more than a year, before the diagnosis is made. In others, the symptoms appear suddenly. Both groups may have had intestinal inflammation for days, months, or even longer, although they may not have experienced symptoms for most of that time.

Will I have to live with IBD for the rest of my life?

As this book goes to print, both Crohn's disease and ulcerative colitis are considered chronic illnesses, which means that you will have the disease for the rest of your life. Medication can reduce the inflammation that is causing symptoms. When inflammation is reduced, the tissue can heal, and you can achieve remission (disappearance of any signs of disease).

Is there a cure for Crohn's disease or ulcerative colitis?

At this time, there is no medical or surgical cure for Crohn's disease, although ulcerative colitis is considered to be cured with surgery.

How will IBD affect my day-to-day life?

The goal of your health care team is to allow your day-to-day life to continue without interruption. You should be able to attend school and activities outside school, go to work, and have a normal life.

Is this disease going to change what I can or can't eat or drink?

Changes in your diet may be necessary to relieve symptoms such as stomach pain or loose bowel movements (diarrhea). Discuss your diet with the doctors and nurses who help take care of you. Foods affect each of us differently, so it is important to pay attention to what foods bother your stomach and avoid them in the future.

I play sports. Will IBD affect my ability to play?

No. Playing sports is important for bone development. There are many professional athletes with IBD. Crohn's disease, however, as well as some medications such as steroids, when taken for many months, can weaken the bones. Your doctor may want you to have a DEXA scan (an x-ray measure of bone strength) before you begin playing contact sports such as football or soccer.

Will IBD affect my social life?

We hope that having IBD will not affect your social life. It is up to you to decide whether you tell your friends about your illness. It is always helpful to have allies who can provide you with support if you should need it.

How did I get IBD in the first place?

We still don't know the cause of either form of IBD. Development of this disease is surely a complex process involving genetics, the immune system, and something in the environment. According to the current theory, the genes you inherited are vulnerable to something in the environment. This environmental factor acts as a trigger, causing your immune system to attack the digestive tract. Once the immune system is switched on, it does not recognize the signal to turn off the attack at the correct time. This results in ongoing tissue damage and causes the symptoms of IBD.

Did I do something to cause this?

The answer is a resounding no. Your actions did not cause this disease.

Where can I find out more information?

There are organizations that can provide very helpful fact-based information (see chapter 22). Remember: the Internet is a useful resource, but read with caution—there are many, many Web sites out there, and not all of the information available is based in fact.

Are there many other people who have IBD?

It is estimated that more than 1 million Americans have inflammatory bowel disease. It occurs in people of all ages. Both Crohn's disease and ulcerative colitis commonly develop in teenagers and young adults. About 10 percent of those affected by IBD are under 18 years of age (100,000 people in the United States).

How will my life change because I have this disease?

You will probably need to take medication daily. You will require more appointments with your doctor than before you had this diagnosis. You may need to stay in the hospital at some point, but most people with IBD are never hospitalized.

Can this disease trigger any other health problems?

Various other problems are, at times, associated with IBD. These can include eye, liver, joint, and skin problems; kidney stones; mouth ulcers; fevers; and sores around your bottom.

Do I have to have surgery?

Medication is the main treatment for people with IBD. Some patients, however, will require surgery over time. There is a place for surgery in treating Crohn's disease and ulcerative colitis. Surgery may be necessary in CD to remove narrowed areas of intestine (strictures) that can cause blockages, or areas of severe disease that do not respond to treatments. It may also be necessary to remove fistulas—abnormal connections between loops of intestines or between intestines and other organs—or to drain abscesses (pockets of pus), if they develop.

In UC, surgery to remove the large intestine will eliminate or cure the disease. Surgery can be considered if severe symptoms do not respond to medical treatments, or if serious complications develop.

Do I have to be hooked up to any equipment?

Most people do not need any special equipment.

How do you treat IBD?

IBD is treated with medications, dietary changes, and, in some cases, surgery.

Is this disease genetic? Am I going to pass it on to my kids?

Genetics research has discovered more than 150 genes associated with Crohn's disease and ulcerative colitis. We know that some families have several members with IBD, but some people with IBD have no family history. There is a genetic link, but what it means at this point remains unclear. Children born to parents who have IBD have a slightly increased risk of developing IBD, but this risk is small.

Will IBD cause me pain?

Abdominal pain, rectal pain, and joint pain are symptoms associated with IBD. These symptoms can usually be controlled by the medications and other treatments prescribed by your doctor.

What are the symptoms of IBD?

Diarrhea, weight loss, and abdominal pain are the most common symptoms for children with Crohn's disease. Blood in the stool, lack of appetite, fevers, joint pain, sores on the skin, and redness of the whites of the eye are less common symptoms. Some children also have trouble gaining weight and growing, even when they do not have many other obvious symptoms.

Ulcerative colitis usually causes crampy abdominal pain and bloody diarrhea. Decreased appetite and weight loss occur when the illness is active, but poor growth in height is rare.

Will the medications make me feel different?

Most medications improve patients' symptoms and make them feel better. But medications can, at times, cause side effects. For example, prednisone (a steroid) may make you moody—down on some days, happy on others. It will also make you very hungry. Methotrexate (a medicine that modifies the immune system) may cause nausea the day after you take it. Mesalamine (an anti-inflammatory) may cause headaches, which will disappear when the dose of the medication is reduced.

Is my IBD going to get worse or better over time?

Both Crohn's disease and ulcerative colitis have periods of quiet (remission), when you feel fine, and periods of activity (flares), when your symptoms are active. It is impossible to predict how you will feel, but the goals of your treatment are to decrease the inflammation, heal the damaged tissue, and make you feel well, giving you the best quality of life possible.

*Can I take care of my condition by myself, or do I need
my mother, father, or guardian to help?*

Younger children need their parents to make sure they are taking their medicines and eating well. As you get older, you will need to be responsible for your medications and for taking good care of yourself in general. This includes getting enough sleep and eating well. You will be able to lead an independent and productive life on your own when the time comes.

*What's going to happen if I do eat or drink something
that I shouldn't?*

Different people react differently, but in general, you might get abdominal pain or loose bowel movements.

*How bad is my case in comparison to other people
who have this condition?*

Everyone is different. It is best not to compare yourself to others.

*How often will I feel fine, compared to the times
I am in pain or uncomfortable?*

There is no way to predict how you will feel. With appropriate treatment, we hope that you will feel well most of the time.

*This whole endoscopy thing doesn't sound very appealing.
Is it really necessary that I do this, and if so, how often?*

A colonoscopy (endoscopic examination of the colon) is necessary to make the diagnosis of Crohn's disease or ulcerative colitis. An upper endoscopy is needed when you have symptoms that suggest inflammation in your esophagus (food pipe), stomach, or small intestine. You will need these tests when the doctor is first finding out why you have been feeling bad. After you have started treatments, there may be circumstances when you will need to have the tests again, to help the doctor understand how your treatments are working. There is no fixed schedule for these tests, but after you have been diagnosed for eight or nine years, you will probably need to undergo a colonoscopy every few years to make sure no complications are developing.

Will I need any other uncomfortable tests or treatments?

An upper GI series or abdominal magnetic resonance imaging (MRI)—imaging studies that require you to drink contrast solutions—is usually necessary to make a picture of the intestines so the doctor can see whether there is inflammation. You may also need other tests that are uncomfortable. These will be explained to you at the time you need them so that you know what to expect.

▣ Appendix

A Guide to IBD Medications

This appendix lists medications that can be used to treat Crohn's disease and ulcerative colitis, alphabetized by their generic names. Every medicine has an approved generic name, which is the chemical name of the drug. When a medication is made by more than one company, each company gives it a unique brand (trade) name, under which the company sells and advertises the medicine. Although the brand name is usually printed most clearly on the packaging, the generic name always appears somewhere on the packaging as well. Please note that this list, including the brand names and dosage forms, is not all inclusive and cannot be kept up to date because new medications may come into the market and older medications may be discontinued or have a change in formulations. You should always speak with your medical team to receive the most up-to-date information about the medications your child is prescribed.

Common IBD medications

Generic name	Brand (trade) name	Dosage forms	Medication class
6-Mercaptopurine	Purinethol	Tablet (50 mg)	Immunomodulator
Adalimumab	Humira, Amjevita	Injection (10, 20, 40 mg injectable solutions)	Biologic agent
Azathioprine	Imuran, Azasan	Tablet (25, 50, 75 mg)	Immunomodulator
Balsalazide	Colazal	Capsule (750 mg)	5-ASA
Budesonide	Entocort EC, Uceris	Capsule (3, 9 mg)	Corticosteroid
Certolizumab pegol	Cimzia	Injection (200 mg)	Biologic agent
Ciprofloxacin	Cipro	Capsule (250, 500 mg)	Antibiotic
Cyclosporine	Neoral, Sandimmune	Capsule (25, 100 mg); liquid (100 mg/mL)	Immunomodulator
Golimumab	Simponi	Injection (50, 100 mg)	Biologic agent

Generic name	Brand (trade) name	Dosage forms	Medication class
Hydrocortisone	Anusol-HC ointment, Anusol-HC suppository, Cortenema, Cortifoam, Proctofoam-HC	Ointment (1%, 2.5%); suppository (25 mg); enema (100 mg/ 60 mL); rectal foam (10%); rectal foam (1%)	Corticosteroid
Infliximab	Remicade, Inflectra	Intravenous powder (100 mg)	Biologic agent
Lansoprazole	Prevacid	Capsule (15, 30 mg); liquid (3 mg/mL)	Acid blocker
Mesalamine	Apriso, Asacol HD, Delzicol, Lialda, Pentasa, Canasa, Rowasa	Tablet, capsule (250, 375, 400, 500, 800 mg; 1.2 g); suppository (500 mg, 1 g); enema (1 g)	5-ASA
Methotrexate	Folex, Mexate, Rheumatrex	Tablet (2.5 mg); injection (25 mg/mL)	Immunomodulator
Methylprednisolone	Medrol	Tablet (2, 4, 8, 16, 32 mg)	Corticosteroid
Metronidazole	Flagyl	Tablet (250, 500 mg); capsule (375 mg)	Antibiotic
Olsalazine	Dipentum	Tablet (250 mg)	5-ASA
Omeprazole	Prilosec	Capsule (10, 20 mg)	Acid blocker
Prednisolone	Pediapred, Prelone	Liquid (5 mg/5 mL; 15 mg/5 mL)	Corticosteroid
Prednisone	Deltasone	Tablet (2.5, 5, 10, 20 mg)	Corticosteroid
Ranitidine	Zantac	Tablet (150 mg); liquid (15 mg/mL)	Acid blocker
Rifaximin	Xifaxin	Tablet (200, 550 mg)	Antibiotic
Sulfasalazine	Azulfidine	Tablet (500 mg)	5-ASA
Tacrolimus	Prograf, Protopic	Capsule (0.5, 1, 5 mg); ointment (0.03%, 0.1%)	Immunomodulator
Thalidomide	Thalomid	Capsule (50, 100, 150, 250 mg)	Immunomodulator
Ustekinumab	Stelara	Intravenous powder (130 mg); injection (90 mg injectable solution)	Biologic agent
Vedolizumab	Entyvio	Intravenous powder (300 mg)	Biologic agent

Glossary

These are common terms and abbreviations you might see or hear in either the doctor's office or the hospital. *Italicized* words in the definition are also defined in this glossary.

Abscess: A "pocket" of pus in the body, caused by infection

Albumin: A protein that is measured in blood tests; an albumin level is a good indicator of inflammation (low levels suggest increased inflammation)

Anastomosis: The process of surgically joining two hollow organs, often after the tissue originally joining them has been surgically removed (*resected*)

Anemia: Lower than normal amounts of *hemoglobin* in the red cells of the blood

Ankylosing spondylitis: A form of joint inflammation primarily involving the spine and the lower back, sometimes seen in patients with IBD

Antibody tests: Blood tests that are sometimes used by doctors to explore whether a patient may have Crohn's disease or ulcerative colitis (These tests are not considered definitive in making a diagnosis of IBD and are not a substitute for imaging studies and endoscopy)

Anus: The opening through which stool (a bowel movement) leaves the body

Arthralgia: Pains in the joints, frequently felt by persons with IBD

Arthritis: Inflammation (swelling) of a joint, accompanied by pain, heat, or redness

5-ASA (5-aminosalicylic acid): Another name for the active component of *mesalamine*, olsalazine, balsalazide, and sulfasalazine

Aseptic necrosis: A complication of the long-term use of high-dose steroids, in which part of a joint (usually the hip) collapses

Autoimmunity: An inflammatory reaction to one's own tissues

Barium: A white chalky substance that helps show parts of the *GI tract* on an x-ray

Barium enema (BE): An x-ray exam of the *colon* and *rectum*, after liquid *barium* has been given to the patient through the *anus*

BID: Abbreviation for twice a day (Latin: *bis in die*)

Biopsy: A small piece of tissue taken from an area of the body and checked under a microscope

BP: Abbreviation for blood pressure

C&S: Abbreviation for culture and sensitivity, a test for bacteria in blood and urine samples

CAT scan: See *CT scan*

CBC: Abbreviation for complete blood count, a type of blood test

CD: Abbreviation for *Crohn's disease*

Celiac disease: An intolerance to gluten (a protein found in rye, barley, and oats), which causes inflammation of the small intestine and symptoms that can mimic those of Crohn's disease

Colectomy: Removal of part or all of the *colon*

Colitis: Inflammation of the large intestine

Colon: The large intestine

Colonoscopy: A test in which a flexible lighted tube is inserted through the *rectum* to examine the large intestine

Colostomy: An opening, created through surgery, that connects the large intestine to the outside of the body through the skin of the abdomen (belly area); stool leaves the body through this opening into a special bag, called an appliance

Comprehensive metabolic panel (CMP): Twelve blood tests that are run from a single blood sample, so that only one blood draw is needed

C-reactive protein (CRP): A blood test that measures inflammation; this protein may be elevated in cases of active IBD

Crohn's disease (CD): A chronic disease that causes inflammation in the esophagus, stomach, small intestine, or large intestine (*colon*)

CT scan: Abbreviation for computed tomography scan, a special type of x-ray

CXR: Abbreviation for chest x-ray

Cytokine: A protein released by cells of the immune system that helps cells "talk" to one another; when produced in excess, some cytokines cause inflammation

Digestive tract: The *gastrointestinal tract*

Discharge summary: A summary, dictated by the doctor during or after a patient's hospital stay, that includes any tests or operations performed, laboratory data, the patient's condition when leaving the hospital, and plans for follow-up care

Distal: Away from the center or away from the beginning; in the *GI tract*, a distal point would be close to the *anus*

Distension: An uncomfortable swelling in the abdomen, often caused by excessive amounts of gas and fluids in the intestine

Dx: Abbreviation for diagnosis

Dysplasia: Changes in cells that may predict the development of cancer

ECG (EKG): Abbreviation for electrocardiogram, the measurement of the electrical activity of the heart

Edema: Accumulation of too much fluid in the tissues, resulting in swelling

Electrolytes: Chemicals, such as salts, that are necessary for the body to keep working

Elemental diet: A specially prepared liquid meal that does not contain any foods to which people typically have a reaction

Endoscopy: The examination of the inside of a hollow organ, such as the intestines, using special lighted tubes

E. nodosum: Abbreviation for *Erythema nodosum*, a skin rash

Enteral nutrition: Delivering food and nutrients into the stomach and intestine, often using a *nasogastric tube*

Enterocyte: Absorptive cell in the *intestinal epithelium*

Episcleritis: Inflammation of the eye, sometimes seen in patients with IBD

Erythema nodosum: Reddish purple swellings, sometimes seen on the lower legs during flares of Crohn's disease and ulcerative colitis

Erythrocyte sedimentation rate (ESR): A blood test that can point to an inflammatory condition in the body; may be increased in active Crohn's disease and ulcerative colitis

Exacerbation: A worsening of symptoms; a relapse; a flare; a period of active disease

Excision: Surgical removal

Extraintestinal manifestations: Inflammation of organ systems other than intestines (skin, joints, eye) sometimes seen in patients with IBD

Exudate: A whitish material seen in an inflamed colon, usually consisting of mucus and white blood cells (pus)

Febrile: Running a fever

Fissure: A crack in the skin; with Crohn's disease, usually near the area of the *anus*

Fistula: An abnormal connection between two locations in the body; for example, the connection can be between loops of intestine, or between the intestine and another structure, such as the bladder, vagina, or skin

Folic acid: One of the vitamins responsible for the maintenance of red blood cells

Fulminant: Disease that develops extremely quickly

Gastroenterologist: A doctor specially trained in the diagnosis and treatment of patients with stomach and intestinal disease

Gastroesophageal reflux (GER): The regurgitation of stomach acid and food back into the esophagus, often causing heartburn or vomiting

Gastrointestinal tract (GI tract): The digestive system, extending from the stomach to the *anus* and including the small and large intestine

Granuloma: A characteristic inflammatory reaction that can be seen in some persons with Crohn's disease

Gut: General word for intestine or bowel

H&P: Abbreviation for *history and physical examination*

Hct: Abbreviation for *hematocrit*

Hematocrit: A measure of the percentage of red blood cells in whole blood (patients with *anemia* have low levels of hematocrit)

Hemoglobin: The part of red blood cells that carries oxygen; low levels of hemoglobin result in *anemia*

Hemorrhage: Abnormally heavy bleeding

Hemorrhoids: Painful, enlarged veins of the lower *rectum* and *anus*, sometimes seen as a complication in people with IBD

Hgb: Abbreviation for *hemoglobin*

History and physical examination (H&P): A record that contains a person's medical history, as well as results from physical exams

HPI: Abbreviation for history of present illness

Hygiene hypothesis: The theory that growing up in a cleaner environment with fewer infections may increase the risk of autoimmune diseases like diabetes and IBD

Hyperalimentation: A way of giving patients additional nutrition (food) through a vein, if they cannot get all their body's dietary needs through eating; also known as *parenteral nutrition* (PN) or *total parenteral nutrition* (TPN)

IBD: Abbreviation for *inflammatory bowel disease*

IBS: Abbreviation for *irritable bowel syndrome*

Idiopathic: Of unknown cause

Ileal pouch–anal anastomosis (IPAA): An operation (also known as the pull-through) for ulcerative colitis, in which an internal pouch is created after a *colectomy*; because the *rectum* is not removed, the patient continues to pass stool through the *anus*

Ileitis: Inflammation of the lower part of the small intestine, seen commonly in Crohn's disease

Ileocecal valve: The border between the end of the small intestine and the beginning of the large intestine

Ileostomy: An opening, created through surgery, that connects the *ileum* to the outside of the body through the skin of the abdomen (belly area); stool leaves the body through this opening into a special bag, called an appliance

Ileum: The lower third of the small intestine, closest to the *colon*

Ileus: Temporary paralysis of the bowel, often resulting from surgery, abdominal infection, or *electrolyte* imbalance

IM: Abbreviation for intramuscular, meaning "into a muscle"

Immunology: Study of the body's immune response to disease

Immunomodulators: Drugs that suppress (hold back) or strengthen the body's immune response

Incontinence: In IBD, the inability to keep stool in the body (resulting in accidents), usually because the *rectum* is inflamed

Indeterminate colitis: A term used to categorize IBD when the distinction between ulcerative colitis and Crohn's disease is unclear

Induction treatment: Using medications to treat a flare and get a sick patient well

Inflammatory bowel disease (IBD): A collective term for Crohn's disease and ulcerative colitis

Intestinal epithelium: Lining of the small intestine

Intractable: Not helped by medical treatments

Irritable bowel syndrome (IBS): Abdominal discomfort, sometimes mistakenly called "spastic colitis"; this condition does not cause inflammation of the *colon* and has no relationship to IBD, but people can have both IBD and IBS

IV: Abbreviation for intravenous, meaning into a vein

KUB: Kidneys, ureters, and bladder; an abdominal x-ray is sometimes called by this name

Lactose breath test: A test that involves drinking a liquid rich in milk sugar (lactose); breath samples are then taken over a period to determine whether there is enough lactase (an enzyme that breaks down milk sugar) in the body

Lactose intolerance (or lactase deficiency): A condition caused by a decrease or absence of the enzyme lactase, which aids in the breakdown of lactose (milk sugar)

Laparoscopy: Surgical procedure in which instruments are inserted into the abdomen through several small openings, leaving several very small scars

Laparotomy (or open surgery): A surgery requiring one large abdominal incision

Left-sided colitis: A form of ulcerative colitis in which only a portion of the colon (the rectum, sigmoid, and descending colon) is inflamed

Leukocytosis: An increased number of white blood cells in blood circulation; a sign of infection

Lumen (intestinal): The hollow area inside the intestine where food and liquid pass through

Magnetic resonance imaging (MRI): An imaging study using magnets (not radiation or x-rays) to show the appearance of organs inside the body

Maintenance therapies (or maintenance treatment): Medications taken when a patient with IBD has the disease under control, to prevent flares

Mesalamine: The generic name for a 5-ASA drug, used to treat inflamed intestine with few, if any, side effects

Motility: In the digestive tract, movement of the muscles that propel food through the intestines

MRI: Abbreviation for *magnetic resonance imaging*

Mucus: In the digestive tract, a clear or whitish substance produced by the intestine, which may be found in the stool

Nasogastric tube (NG tube): A thin, flexible tube passed through the nose in order to remove liquids and air that collect in the stomach, when the bowel is obstructed or after intestinal surgery, or to deliver nutrients (food) into the stomach

NPO: Abbreviation for nothing by mouth (Latin: *nil per os*)

Obstruction: In the digestive tract, a blockage of the small or large intestine that prevents the normal passage of intestinal contents

Occult blood: Hidden blood in the stool, often an indication of disease activity; simple lab tests can determine the presence of occult blood

Operative report: A complete record of an operation, dictated by the surgeon after surgery

Ostomy: An artificial opening made surgically

Pancolitis: Ulcerative colitis that involves the entire large intestine; the most common type of ulcerative colitis found in children

Parenteral nutrition (PN): Delivering nutrients (including carbohydrates, fat, and proteins) directly into a vein to provide nutrition to people who cannot take enough food into their stomach or intestines

Pathogen: A bacterium or virus that causes disease

Pathogenesis: The origin and development of disease

Pathology report: Results of examining tissues removed from the body during surgery or *biopsy*

Peptic ulcers: Erosions in the lining of the stomach or duodenum (first part of the small intestine)

Percutaneous endoscopic gastrostomy (PEG): Using an endoscope to place a feeding tube into the stomach

Perforation: A hole in an organ; in the digestive tract, a perforation is usually a hole in the bowel wall, allowing what is inside the intestines to spill into the abdominal cavity

Perianal: The area around the anal opening; this area may become inflamed and irritated in persons with Crohn's disease

Peristalsis: The normal regular movements of the stomach and intestines

Peristomal: The area immediately surrounding the *stoma*

Peritonitis: Inflammation of the peritoneum (the membrane enclosing the abdominal organs); peritonitis usually results from an intestinal *perforation* or infection

Pharynx: Throat

Plt: Abbreviation for platelet count

PO: Abbreviation for by mouth (Latin: *per os*)

Polygenic: Caused by multiple inherited genes

Polyp: A small growth in the intestine; in young children, polyps can cause rectal bleeding but are almost never cancerous

Pouchitis: Inflammation of the ileoanal pouch (a pouch created by a surgical procedure performed in patients with ulcerative colitis)

Primary sclerosing cholangitis (PSC): An autoimmune disease that causes scarring of the bile ducts, leading to fatigue and jaundice (yellow skin)

PRN: Abbreviation for as needed (Latin: *pro re nata*)

Proctectomy: Surgical removal of the *rectum*

Proctitis: Inflammation of the *rectum*

Proctocolectomy: Removal of the entire *colon* and *rectum*

Progress notes: A daily record of a hospitalized patient's progress, test results, and so forth, completed by the professionals who care for the patient

Prolapse: The falling, or protrusion (pushing forward), of an organ

Proximal: Closer to the beginning; in the digestive tract, a proximal point is closer to the mouth

PSC: Abbreviation for primary sclerosing cholangitis

Pyoderma gangrenosum: A type of sore or ulcer that sometimes occurs on the arms or legs of persons with IBD

Q4H: Abbreviation for every 4 hours

QD: Abbreviation for every day

QID: Abbreviation for four times per day

QOD: Abbreviation for every other day

RAP: Abbreviation for recurrent abdominal pain

RBC: Abbreviation for *red blood cell*

Rectum: The part of the intestine that connects the *colon* to the *anus*

Regional enteritis: A name for Crohn's disease affecting the small intestine

Remission: A lessening of symptoms and a return to good health

Resection: Surgical removal

Reservoir: A surgically created pouch that collects waste

RX: Abbreviation for prescription or therapy (medications)

S: Abbreviation for without (Latin: *sans*)

Sacroiliitis: Inflammation of the large joints where the spine meets the pelvis in the lower back

SBFT: Abbreviation for small bowel follow-through, used when describing an upper GI x-ray in which *barium* is followed all the way through the entire small intestine (see also *upper GI series*)

SED rate (or sedimentation rate): See *erythrocyte sedimentation rate*

Short bowel syndrome: A condition in which so much diseased bowel has been surgically removed that the remaining intestine can no longer absorb sufficient nutrients

Sigmoidoscopy: A test in which a lighted tube is passed through the *rectum* into the part of the *colon* nearest to it

Small bowel: Small intestine

Spastic colon: An old, obsolete term sometimes used to describe *irritable bowel syndrome*

Sphincter: A ring of muscle tissue that keeps closed certain parts of the digestive tract (like the *anus*)

Stenosis: A narrowing of an area

Stoma: A surgically created opening of the bowel through the skin in the abdomen

Stricture: Narrowing; in IBD, a narrowed area of intestine caused by active inflammation or scar tissue

Strictureplasty: A surgical procedure that widens narrowed areas of intestine (*strictures*)

Subtotal colectomy: Removal of part or most of the *colon*, leaving a part (usually the *rectum*) intact

Sutures: Materials used in surgery to close wounds

Tenesmus: A constant urge to empty the bowel (pass stool), usually caused by inflammation of the *rectum*

TID: Abbreviation for three times a day

Total parenteral nutrition (TPN): See *hyperalimentation*

Toxic megacolon: Severe dilation (enlargement) of the *colon* in ulcerative colitis (or occasionally in Crohn's disease), which may lead to *perforation*

TPR: Abbreviation for temperature, pulse, and respiration

Transmural inflammation: Inflammation involving the whole thickness of the intestinal wall, seen in Crohn's disease but not in ulcerative colitis

Tx: Abbreviation for treatment

Ulcerative colitis (UC): A chronic disease that causes inflammation of the large intestine

Ulcerative proctitis: A form of ulcerative colitis in which only the rectum is inflamed

Ultrasound: An imaging study using sound waves to show the appearance of organs inside the body

Upper endoscopy (esophagogastroduodenoscopy, EGD): Examination with a camera of the esophagus, stomach, and duodenum

Upper GI series (UGI): An x-ray exam of the esophagus, stomach, and duodenum (first part of the small intestine) performed in patients after they drink liquid *barium*; when the exam is made longer to allow the barium to go through the entire small intestine, the x-ray is then known as an upper GI series with small bowel follow-through (see *SBFT*)

US or U/S: Abbreviation for *ultrasound*

Uveitis: Inflammation of the eye sometimes seen in IBD

Villi: Fingerlike projections containing absorptive cells that line the intestine and help in the digestion and absorption of food

WBC: Abbreviation for *white blood cell*

Within normal limits (WNL): A term used to describe a laboratory test result that is similar to results seen in healthy people

X-ray reports: Results of x-ray studies (tests)

Index

Page numbers in *italics* indicate figures and tables.

About the North American Society for Pediatric Gastroenterology, Hepatology and Nutrition (NASPGHAN) and the NASPGHAN Foundation

NASPGHAN

Mission

NASPGHAN's mission is to advance the understanding of normal development, physiology, and pathophysiology of diseases of the gastrointestinal (GI) tract and liver in children; improve quality of care by fostering the dissemination of this knowledge through scientific meetings, professional and public education, and policy development; and serve as an effective voice for members and the profession.

The membership of NASPGHAN consists of more than 1,500 pediatric gastroenterologists, in the United States, Puerto Rico, Mexico, and Canada.

NASPGHAN strives to improve the care of infants, children, and adolescents with digestive disorders by promoting advances in clinical care, research, and education. Pediatric gastroenterologists specialize in the care of many gastrointestinal conditions in children, including chronic abdominal pain, diarrhea, constipation, vomiting, GI tract bleeding, inflammatory bowel disease, liver diseases, diseases of the pancreas, poor weight gain, and nutritional problems. Pediatric gastroenterologists can perform a number of diagnostic and treatment procedures, such as upper endoscopy, colonoscopy, liver biopsies, placement of feeding tubes into the stomach, control of gastrointestinal bleeding, and manometry (or pressure) studies of the esophagus, colon, and rectum.

Objectives

NASPGHAN's objectives include but are not limited to:
Improving the digestive health and nutrition of children worldwide and
  particularly in North America
Fostering dialogue and research on pertinent issues that affect pediatric
  gastroenterology patients and their families
Providing opportunities for clinicians and researchers to gain knowledge
  of the scientific advances in the field of pediatric gastroenterology
Disseminating the wealth of existing scientific information to improve clinical
  outcomes and advance the practice of pediatric gastroenterology and
  nutrition

NASPGHAN Foundation

Mission

To fund and promote research and educational programs that will advance the creation, application, and dissemination of knowledge of gastrointestinal, hepatobiliary, pancreatic, and nutritional disorders in children.

To identify, encourage, support, and coordinate scientific research and professional study of these pediatric disorders.

To strengthen the role of pediatric gastrointestinal and nutritional scientists as leaders in research and education in these medical and health care fields.

To evaluate and improve the quality and availability of medical care for children with digestive disorders.

To support the research and educational programs of NASPGHAN.

Objective

NASPGHAN Foundation has a single goal: to improve the treatment and management of gastrointestinal, hepatobiliary, pancreatic, and nutritional disorders in children. Through our work, we provide information and resources to parents, patients, and medical professionals dealing with these disorders.

The NASPGHAN Foundation promotes research, education, and awareness of pediatric digestive and nutritional disorders.